The Trans Fat
SOLUTION

Cooking and Shopping to Eliminate
the Deadliest Fat from Your Diet

Kim Severson

with Cindy Burke

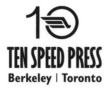

TEN SPEED PRESS
Berkeley | Toronto

1⊖

Ten Speed Press
Box 7123
Berkeley, California 94707
www.tenspeed.com

Distributed in Australia by Simon & Schuster Australia, in Canada by Ten Speed Press Canada, in New Zealand by Southern Publishers Group, in South Africa by Real Books, and in the United Kingdom and Europe by Airlift Book Company.

Cover and text design by Catherine Jacobes
Cover photograph by Jonathan Chester
Photo of Kim Severson on page 126 by Mike Kepka
Photo of Cindy Burke on page 126 by Adrian Lee Photography

Library of Congress Cataloging-in-Publication Data
Severson, Kim.
   The trans fat solution : cooking and shopping to eliminate the deadliest fat from your diet / Kim Severson with Cindy Burke.
       p. cm.
Includes bibliographical references and index.
   ISBN 1-58008-543-1
   1. Lipids in human nutrition. 2. Trans fatty acids. I. Burke, Cindy.
II. Title.
   TX553.L5S48 2003
   613.2'84--dc22

                                        2003017443

Printed in Canada
First printing, 2003

2 3 4 5 6 7 8 9 10 — 07 06 05 04 03

CONTENTS

ACKNOWLEDGMENTS

Thanks first to Michael Bauer and Miriam Morgan, my editors at the *San Francisco Chronicle* and the pair who encouraged my initial interest in this subject. They and the entire Food staff at the *Chronicle* offer daily encouragement, inspiration, and a good knock in the head when I need it. Thanks, too, to my agent Amy Rennert; our fine editor at Ten Speed, Julie Bennett; and Professor Marion Nestle, for her brainy science consultations. A big high five to Cindy Burke, my best friend and an amazing cook. And last, thanks to my mother, Anne Severson, who loves to cook, and my father, Jim Severson, who loves to eat.

—Kim Severson

My daughter Allison awakened my desire to create healthy alternatives for foods she enjoyed. Thanks to my partner, Pat, my friends, and my family for praise and encouragement as they tasted their way through many of these recipes. Thanks also to chefs Madeleine Kamman and Barbara Figueroa for teaching me to pay attention to details, take notes, and taste everything—twice. Special thanks to my dear friend Kim Severson for sharing this opportunity. Our mutual delight in food and cooking has made this book a pleasure to write.

—Cindy Burke

PREFACE

I write about food for a daily newspaper in San Francisco. When it comes to eating, our newsroom is like any other in the nation. If there's food around and a hungry reporter is on deadline, the food will get eaten. Cold pizza, stale cookies—leave it out and sometime between reporting a story and putting the paper to bed, someone will wolf it down. In the Food department, where we like to think our culinary standards are a little higher, we joke that you could leave out a hammer covered in chocolate frosting and it would be gone by morning—especially if you leave it in the Sports department.

That's why I was surprised one day when a sports reporter came by my desk with a popular breakfast bar in hand. He wanted to know if it was made with trans fat.

I had been writing about trans fat, a processed substance that is laced throughout most Americans' diets. Think Crisco or a stick of margarine, and you've got trans fat—more formally called trans fatty acid. Eat an average-size order of fast-food fries, and you've just consumed several grams of it. The stuff is worse for your arteries than a cup of beef tallow. Researchers are gathering an increasingly large body of evidence that shows trans fat can change the way cells behave—for the worse—clogging the body's biological workings. Some suspect it can cause cancer and speed the onset of diabetes. According to the Food and Drug Administration's (FDA) own research, listing information about trans fat on nutrition labels could prevent 7,600 to 17,100 cases of coronary heart disease and 2,500 to 5,600 deaths every year. Not only would people be able to choose more healthful foods, but some manufacturers would choose to reduce trans fat amounts rather than list high levels on nutrition labels.

But trans fat is incredibly useful to food manufacturers because it's a relatively inexpensive way to make crackers and piecrusts crisp, and it extends the shelf life of baked goods. It's a key ingredient in everything from microwave popcorn to Coffee Mate. By the FDA's estimate, more than 40 percent of the food on grocery store shelves has trans fat.

The problem is, it's difficult to know when you're eating it—even if you try to avoid the obvious suspects like supermarket bakery cakes, mass-marketed salty snacks, and fast-food french fries. Trans fat is only beginning to be listed on the nutrition labels of food packaging, and it hides in places most people would never suspect: cereal, frozen waffles, premium ice cream, peanut butter, and even lowfat cookies and seemingly healthy energy bars. Unless you know some tricks to reading a label, there's no way to tell. In July 2003, the FDA finally ordered manufacturers to list trans fat amounts on nutrition labels, but the rule doesn't take effect until 2006. Although some companies are starting to list trans fat amounts on packaging, shoppers will have to fend for themselves for a few more years.

As always, consumers are way ahead of government regulators. Concern about trans fat—and more widely about the way our food is processed—is becoming so prevalent that even a newspaper sports writer, hungry and on deadline, would pause long enough to question what he was about to eat. I showed him how to read the label. We figured out that the breakfast bar did contain a couple of grams of trans fat. He ate it anyway, but at least he was able to make an informed choice.

This book is for him and others like him who want to avoid trans fat. We don't intend to be preachy or overly scientific—there's no faster way to take the joy out of eating. We're not the food militia, nor do we intend to suggest you give up fat or snacking. Rather, we offer a readable guide to trans fat coupled with some easy-to-understand tips on how to figure out if the food you're about to buy is full of the stuff. Then we take things one step further, offering straightforward, good-tasting recipes to replace the convenience foods that are often high in trans fat—foods like frozen toaster waffles, fried chicken, jalapeño cheese poppers, potpies, cake mixes, and crackers. And because we just happen to think there isn't anything much more satisfying than a plate of hot french fries, we've included a recipe for a trans fat–free version.

The woman behind most of the recipes is Cindy Burke, a former professional chef who is raising a young daughter. She was skeptical about the project at first, but then she started reading the labels on some of the food she was feeding her child. Granola, fish sticks, crackers—all of them had trans fat. So she went to work creating recipes that would allow her the convenience of packaged foods but offer a much healthier nutritional profile. And frankly, they taste a whole lot better than anything you could buy.

None of this is an attempt to teach the science of fat manufacturing, preach the ills of fat, or bash a government food regulatory system that gives too much leeway to food manufacturers. We put this book together because we couldn't find anything else out there that offered an easy-to-understand guide to the most common but most deadly fat in America. And we wanted to provide some delicious solutions to the trans fat dilemma—whether you're a serious cook or a hungry sports writer.

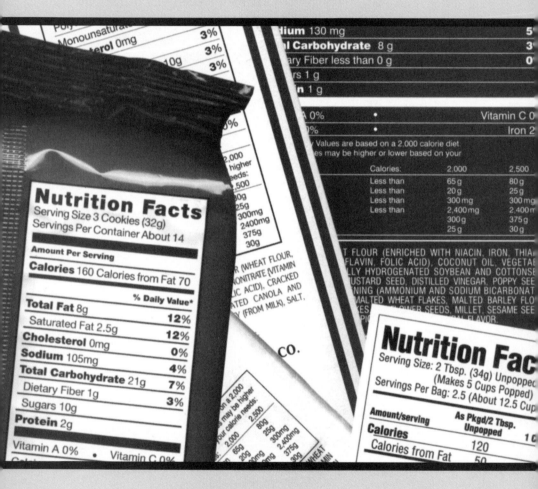

Poly...
Monounsaturated...
...terol 0mg   3%
...10g   3%
                                      3%

Nutrition Facts
Serving Size 3 Cookies (32g)
Servings Per Container About 14

Amount Per Serving

Calories 160 Calories from Fat 70

	% Daily Value*
Total Fat 8g	**12%**
Saturated Fat 2.5g	**12%**
Cholesterol 0mg	**0%**
Sodium 105mg	**4%**
Total Carbohydrate 21g	**7%**
Dietary Fiber 1g	**3%**
Sugars 10g	
Protein 2g	

Vitamin A 0%   •   Vitamin C 0%

...dium 130 mg   5
...l Carbohydrate 8 g   3
...ary Fiber less than 0 g   0
...rs 1 g
...n 1 g

...A 0%   •   Vitamin C 0
...%)   •   Iron 2

...y Values are based on a 2,000 calorie diet.
...es may be higher or lower based on your

	Calories:	2,000	2,500
Less than		65g	80g
Less than		20g	25g
Less than		300 mg	300 mg
Less than		2,400mg	2,400 m
		300g	375g
		25g	30g

...R (WHEAT FLOUR,
...ONITRATE (VITAMIN
...LIC ACID), CRACKED
...ATED CANOLA AND
...Y (FROM MILK), SALT,

...CO.

...T FLOUR (ENRICHED WITH NIACIN, IRON, THIA
...FLAVIN, FOLIC ACID), COCONUT OIL, VEGETA
...LY HYDROGENATED SOYBEAN AND COTTONSE
...USTARD SEED, DISTILLED VINEGAR, POPPY SEE
...NING (AMMONIUM AND SODIUM BICARBONAT
...MALTED WHEAT FLAKES, MALTED BARLEY FLO
...ES, ...OWER SEEDS, MILLET, SESAME SEE
...PI... ...AL FLAVOR.

Nutrition Fac
Serving Size: 2 Tbsp. (34g) Unpopped
(Makes 5 Cups Popped)
Servings Per Bag: 2.5 (About 12.5 Cup

Amount/serving	As Pkgd/2 Tbsp. Unpopped
Calories	1 C
Calories from Fat	50

The Lowdown on the Deadliest Fat in Your Diet

What Exactly Is Trans Fat?

Trans fatty acid, or trans fat for short, might seem like a mind-numbing scientific term, but it's likely you're very familiar with it. In fact, you probably grew up with trans fat on your table, in the form of a stick of margarine. If you've got a can of Crisco in your kitchen cupboard, then you've got trans fat in the house. Called "partially hydrogenated vegetable oil" on food labels, trans fat is the only man-made fat in the food supply. And it is the worst fat you can eat.

"There should be a warning on food made with this stuff like there is on nicotine products. It's that bad for you," said Dr. Jeffrey Aron, a University of California at San Francisco professor of medicine and one of the nation's leading experts on fatty acids and their effects on the body. He is one of a growing body of doctors and dietitians who agree that trans fat is one of the worst food additives in America's diet.

Food manufacturers love trans fat as much as health professionals hate it. Trans fat is an inexpensive way to prolong shelf life and make food smoother, crispier, or softer. Partially hydrogenated oil gives texture to the cream inside an Oreo and that nice crunch to the chocolate cookies that surround it. Crackers like Cheez-Its and even seemingly healthier snacks like baked Wheat Thins get their crispness from trans fat. It's the reason Twinkies stay so soft and fresh on the store shelf for what seems like an eternity, and what makes the frosting on a supermarket cake creamy.

Home cooks love it because it can make a piecrust nearly foolproof or give a piece of fried chicken its crispy coat. And as a component of margarine, trans fat provides an inexpensive, less-saturated alternative to butter. Fast-food operators are equally enamored. Every chicken McNugget at McDonald's, every french fry at Burger King and virtually anything else fried at a fast-food outlet is cooked in oil that contains trans fat. Since the fat is so highly processed, it doesn't break down easily and can stand up to the repeated, high-heat pounding of the fryers in fast-food restaurants.

This creamy, artificial fat is so embedded in the groceries we buy, the restaurant food we eat, and the food we cook at home that it has become virtually invisible—especially because food manufacturers won't be required to list trans fat alongside other kinds of fats on nutritional labels until 2006. But there is almost no escaping it. According to the FDA, nearly half of all cereals, both cold and hot, contain trans fat. So do 70 percent of cake mixes, 75 percent of chips and other salty snacks, 80 percent of frozen breakfast foods like waffles, and nine out of ten cookies. Even the products people buy when they want to eat healthier—granola, lowfat cookies and crackers, and even some power bars—are made with partially hydrogenated vegetable oil. Foods marked "low in cholesterol" or "low in saturated fat" might have high levels of trans fat. So do most major brands of peanut butter. Microwave popcorn is drowning in it—even the brands marked lower fat. During a recent survey I did of 140 varieties of crackers that lined the shelves of a major national supermarket chain, only a handful did not contain partially hydrogenated oil.

Why Does It Make My Piecrust Taste So Good?

As any cook will tell you, there is much to recommend a fat that can stay solid at room temperature. Mixed together in a certain order and in the right amounts, flour plus a solid fat like butter, lard, or shortening are what make croissants flaky and give piecrusts their texture. Fat, especially a solid fat like butter or shortening, is the ingredient needed to make sure flour doesn't develop tough strands of gluten when it's mixed with liquid. Gluten is what makes bread dough springy and elastic. Fat acts like a barrier, preventing the flour molecules from tangling and joining up into strands. Fat also adds flavor and texture. In cakes, fat helps trap the air bubbles that make a cake rise. By preventing the flour proteins from linking to form gluten, fat helps make a cake tender. There are infinite pastry recipes that call for a combination of flour, fat, and liquid. Some require the labor-intensive skill that creates the 729 layers in a classic French puff pastry. Others are based on a simple method of rubbing butter or shortening or lard into flour and rolling it out to create an American-style piecrust.

Melted fat becomes a reliable medium for the griddle or the deep-fat fryer, too. Southern cooks love the crispy result when a piece of chicken is fried in a cast-iron pan full of lard, or the modern-day alternative—Crisco. In fact, Crisco has some practical advantages. Because it is relatively healthy vegetable oil that's been chemically altered to be stable—essentially meaning it doesn't easily go bad—shortening can be heated repeatedly and not burn or go rancid. The flavor is perfectly neutral for cooks who don't want the roasty flavor lard can impart. And, of course, Crisco is a whole lot easier and cheaper to come by than good, rendered lard.

Marion Cunningham, America's champion of home cooking and the woman who revised *The Fannie Farmer Cookbook,* swears by Crisco for piecrusts. She's well aware of the dangers of trans fat, but she thinks the small amount one might consume in a piecrust is well worth the foolproof nature of working with it—especially for cooks without much experience. She explains that cutting butter into flour for a piecrust requires strict attention to temperature. Warm hands and too much mixing can make butter soften or even melt, creating a tough crust devoid of flaky layers. Crisco doesn't melt at body temperature, so the risk of overworking the dough and melting the fat is much less than with butter or even lard. Plus, it's economical, she argues.

"There is no simpler, easier way for a cook to get a flaky piecrust—especially for a beginner," she said. "I will always have a can of Crisco around."

The problem is, an increasingly large body of research shows that partially hydrogenated fat is simply the worst fat you can eat.

How Trans Fat Became America's Fat of Choice

Hydrogenated oils have been around for more than a hundred years, arriving shortly after scientists discovered a process to extract oil from corn, soybeans, and seeds. Although we can hardly imagine cooking without those oils today, at the turn of the nineteenth century liquid fats were useless in a European-based culture where butter and lard were the fats of choice. But then a scientist named William Normann discovered a way to turn that relatively healthy liquid vegetable oil into something that stayed solid at room temperature. His hydrogenation process, patented in 1903, basically shoots hydrogen through hot unsaturated oil until the molecules are saturated with it. The chemical alteration in the fat molecules makes the previously liquid oil stay solid at room temperature. The result is so stable—meaning it won't easily go rancid—that it improves the shelf life of any food made with it. (See "The Science of Hydrogenating Oil.") His discovery became so popular that partially hydrogenated oil quickly became the most widely used solid fat in American food processing. And it would eventually turn an entire butter-eating nation into one that preferred spreading trans fat on its toast. Today, Americans eat an estimated 2,000 percent more trans fat than they did in the early 1900s.

America's home cooks were introduced to partially hydrogenated vegetable oil in 1911, when Crisco came along. At the time, Procter & Gamble called its new product "a scientific discovery which will affect every kitchen." It was cheaper than butter, and at cooking demonstrations around the country, home economists showed that it could perform as well as butter in baking. It was touted as healthier than lard and with broader applications in the kitchen. The company also began selling it in huge barrels to commercial bakeries, restaurants, and hotels. In the 1920s, looking to expand the market, the company began targeting ethnic groups. An early Crisco cookbook was targeted specially to Jewish homemakers. Frying potato pancakes in shortening was pushed as healthier and cheaper than using butter. The company touted the pure vegetable oil as just the ticket for an economical, kosher kitchen. "With its blue and white wrapper with the Hebrew inscription, it is very easy to recognize Crisco—the strictly kosher product," the cookbook reads.

Partially hydrogenated oil didn't really settle in to a comfortable place on the American table until World War II, when people turned to

The Science of Hydrogenating Oil

For all you science geeks, here's a snapshot of the molecular properties of trans fatty acid. Trans fat is made when a relatively healthy polyunsaturated liquid vegetable oil from plants like corn, soybeans, cottonseed, or rapeseed (called canola) is bombarded with hydrogen gas and a metal catalyst, usually nickel or platinum. The process takes several hours and happens at temperatures of between 250° and 410°F.

That's the broad stroke. More specifically, fatty acid molecules are basically chains of carbon atoms. They are set up as double bonds of carbon, with hydrogen atoms linked together and surrounded, or saturated, by hydrogen atoms. In some fatty acids, the carbons are double bonded. Fatty acids with one double bond are called *monounsaturated;* fatty acids with two or more double bonds are called *polyunsaturated.* In unsaturated fatty acids, the hydrogen atoms are on the same side of the carbon chain. The shape matters because fatty acids stack together. Change the shape of any molecule and you change how it stacks and behaves in the body. Naturally saturated fats found in butter and lard have hydrogen atoms on both sides of the carbon chain. They are straight, and therefore pack together tightly. That's why saturated fat stays solid at room temperature.

To make artificial saturated fat—trans fat—the double bonds in unsaturated fat are saturated with hydrogen. But completely flooding the molecules with hydrogen atoms would make the fat too stiff for cooking. That's why manufacturers only partially hydrogenate the oil. Thus, the term "partially hydrogenated" is on food ingredient lists. These new trans fat molecules are sort of freaks of nature—they really don't fit in to the natural cellular makeup—and that's why researchers suspect they cause so many problems in the body.

It's important to note that high-heat processing techniques used to make liquid oils stable and neutral-tasting can create small amounts of trans fat as well. Trans fatty acids form at 320°F, which is far lower than the temperature at which most edible vegetable oils are processed. Also, some small amounts of naturally occurring trans fat can be found in beef and high-fat dairy products like milk because trans fat is produced in the gastrointestinal lining of cattle. That form of trans fat, called conjugated linoleic acid, has a different molecular structure and doesn't do damage to the body in the way artificial trans fat does.

margarine and shortening as alternatives to rationed butter. Statistics on table spread consumption offered by the USDA show that the nation's per capita butter consumption dropped from a high of almost 18 pounds a year in the early 1900s to under 10 pounds a year in 1949. But it was a desire for a healthier diet that really tipped the scales in favor of what would turn out to be the unhealthiest fat of all.

In 1957, the American Heart Association first proposed that modifying dietary fats, especially saturated fats like butter and beef fat, would reduce coronary heart disease. Polyunsaturated fats, like margarine, were the suggested alternatives. Three years later, margarine consumption finally surpassed butter, and each American was eating about 9 pounds a year. Margarine consumption would continue to hold steady through the end of the twentieth century, while butter consumption dropped to about 5 pounds a year, driven by a fear of saturated animal fat. The late 1980s and early 1990s were a particularly lucrative time for companies that manufactured partially hydrogenated oil. The public embraced the connection between heart disease and saturated fats, and banished butter and animal fats from the table. Fast-food restaurants replaced the beef fat in the fryers with partially hydrogenated oils. Products like Snackwell's cookies were introduced in 1993 and a year later, they sold better than two other Nabisco brands: Oreo and Chips Ahoy!

BYE-BYE TROPICS

In a strange twist, healthier coconut and palm oils also fell by the wayside. Once used liberally in food manufacturing, the tropical fats (which stay solid at room temperature and can offer more flavor and texture, ounce for ounce, than trans fat) were villainized. Anyone who needs to be especially concerned about too much saturated fat needs to watch how much of it they eat. But tropical oils behave differently in the body than saturated fats from animals, offering such nutritive value that trans fat looks like rat poison in comparison. For people in many Asian cultures, coconut oil is a healthy mainstay. Some nutritionists now suggest people eat two or three tablespoons a day as a way to boost immune systems and counter the effects of so called "bad fat" in the diet.

But in the 1980s, led by a public health campaign to lower saturated fat in the American diet, tropical oils were drummed out of the market.

The public face was a millionaire heart patient named Phil Sokoloff who took out an ad in the *New York Times* in 1988 that claimed palm and coconut oil were killing him and blamed the government for doing nothing. He was joined by the Center for Science in the Public Interest (CSPI), which would later emerge as one of the leaders in the fight to get trans fat listed on food labels. Although there has never been a solid connection made, proponents of tropical oils blame the soy oil industry, which was intent on quashing competition from Malaysian palm oil manufacturers. Certainly, the American Soybean Association played its part by testifying in front of Congress about the evils of tropical oils. As a result, trans fat consumption rocketed.

THE FAST-FOOD PHENOMENON

Fast food and convenience foods started to hit the market in the late 1960s and '70s, and a key ingredient in everything from TV dinners to french fries was partially hydrogenated oil. Demographic and social changes saw more single-parent families or families with two working parents, which meant less time to cook. Convenience foods and eating out became a bigger part of the American diet. Today, more than a third of all calories are eaten outside the home. Kids eat 40 percent of their meals at fast-food restaurants. But it wasn't just an increase in the frequency of fast-food meals and microwave dinners. Portion sizes increased too, leading to even more trans fat in our bellies. The original order of McDonald's fries weighed in at about two ounces and contained 200 calories. In the 1972, the large order of fries was introduced, which had 320 calories. By the mid-1990s, "super size" was coined and an order of french fries grew to 540 calories and 25 grams of fat, according to CSPI. These larger servings added up to a huge increase in the amount of trans fat people were consuming. Cheap trans fat made it possible for the food industry to produce record amounts of inexpensive, shelf-stable junk food. And, many health experts now agree, this is a key link in the obesity epidemic.

So not only was partially hydrogenated oil a cheaper alternative to butter and perceived to be healthier than other fats, but it also gave food manufacturers another advantage—the fat it contributed to products didn't have to be listed on the nutritional labels. That meant that when the lowfat food boom hit in the late 1980s and consumers were hungry for products like Snackwells cookies and reduced-fat Triscuits, food manufacturers could offer products that had a lower saturated fat listing on nutrition labels without having to include trans fat in the unhealthy "saturated fat" category—even though trans fat acts like saturated fat in the body. The foods were, in fact, lower in overall fat, but the labeling glitch made them seem healthier than they were. So even though consumers saw what looked like lower levels of unhealthy saturated fat, each cookie was still packed with partially hydrogenated oil—albeit lesser amounts than full-fat cookies or crackers.

Why Trans Fat Is So Bad for You

Although mainstream medicine has been coming around to the ills of trans fat since only the late 1990s, suspicions about it started bubbling up in the scientific community in the late 1970s, led by the nation's premier lipid researcher, Mary Enig. The biochemistry professor at the University of Maryland was the first researcher to make a compelling case that trans fatty acids were dangerously different than saturated animal fat, and that instead of being the solution to ridding the American diet of saturated fats, trans fat was doing more harm.

The problems with trans fat are many. Like beef fat, trans fat also raises the level of bad cholesterol (LDL), which can clog the arteries and make them inflexible, leading to strokes and heart attacks. But trans fat takes things one step further, scrubbing away the good cholesterol (HDL) that keeps arteries clean. Trans fat also raises other bad blood lipids that can contribute to heart disease. And it does its work faster. An American Heart Association study released in 2002 showed that food cooked with trans fat clogs arteries quicker than food cooked in animal-based saturated fat. But trans fat has what researchers are beginning to agree is a more insidious function in the body: It actually reprograms how cells work, causing lifelong damage that can lead to diabetes, stroke, and possibly cancer. Unlike saturated fats from animals, trans fats aren't easily broken down in the body. The molecular structure of trans fat is so different, so unnatural, that the body has no way to know exactly how to process it. That's why some doctors, in particular the top nutrition and heart experts at Harvard University, believe trans fat is worse than saturated fat.

EVEN A SMALL AMOUNT CAN DO BIG DAMAGE

Leading the pack is Walter Willett, the Harvard University 〈 turning the USDA food pyramid on its head by changing the dietary fat. He suggests we ban trans fat, limit animal fat, an more of healthy fats like olive oil and canola oil. He is an enemy to big-league food processors everywhere. From his office in Harvard's School of Public Health, Willett oversees the longest-running health studies in the nation, which include almost 250,000 doctors, nurses, and other health professionals who regularly fill out extensive questionnaires about their health and diet. Willett's crew discovered that people who ate a lot of trans fat are 50 percent more likely to develop heart disease than people who eat very little. His ongoing Nurses' Health Study of 80,000 women also showed that for each 2 percent increase in the amount of calories from trans fat, a woman's coronary risk will jump by 93 percent. That's just 2 percent. It's no wonder that the *New England Journal of Medicine* reported in 2002 that for women who want to reduce their risk of heart disease, replacing saturated and trans fats with mono- or polyunsaturated fats is more effective than cutting down on the total amount of fat they eat. "Probably millions of people have died prematurely from all the trans fats that have been included in our diet," Willett said in a 2003 interview with *EatingWell* magazine.

BEYOND HEART DISEASE

A growing number of doctors also believe trans fat plays a starring role in a health crisis more prevalent and possibly more damaging than clogged arteries: Syndrome X. Also called metabolic syndrome or, more commonly, beer belly syndrome, the condition has increased along with the amount of refined foods and partially hydrogenated oil Americans eat. Former Stanford University director of endocrinology Gerald Reaven named Syndrome X in 1988 after he observed a collection of health problems ultimately linked to cells' inability to process insulin. Researchers believe trans fat is one of the reasons cells malfunction. Although trans fat only makes up a small part of the average daily diet—somewhere between 3 to 8 percent of the total daily caloric intake—even a handful of grams a day is enough to gum up the workings of a cell. Dr. Jeffrey M. Aron, coauthor with Harriette E. Aron of *Gut-Check: Your Prime Source for Bowel Health and Colon Cancer Prevention* (1stBooks Library, 2001), explains it like this: Picture the cell as a Swiss watch. Sprinkle a few very fine grains of sand in that watch and it will continue to tick, but after a while it won't keep accurate time. Eventually it won't work. That's how trans fat works in the body, he says. It changes how the cell membranes work—how they talk to each other and function. Trans fat can help make cells resistant to insulin, and when you have resistance to insulin you have obesity, he believes.

In 2002, researchers at the Centers for Disease Control (CDC) released estimates that showed at least 47 million Americans, more than 20 percent, could have Syndrome X. Other Syndrome X experts say that estimate is conservative and put the figure as high as 70 million. If you have a combination of any three of these symptoms—high blood sugar, high blood pressure, high levels of blood fats called triglycerides, high cholesterol, or abdominal obesity—the beer belly—you probably have Syndrome X. People with Syndrome X are likely candidates for diabetes, heart attack, cancer, and even Alzheimer's, says Jack Challem, a Tucson-based nutrition expert who has written extensively on Syndrome X. Challem, coauthor with Burton Berkson of *Syndrome X: The Complete Nutritional Program to Prevent and Reverse Insulin Resistance* (John Wiley & Sons, 2001), says that trans fat is such a hidden part of the American diet, people have no idea what it contributes to their illness. "Forty years after it's been in the food system on such a large scale, what is becoming clear is that this is dangerous stuff," Challen said.

And like many health experts, he's amazed at how prevalent yet how hidden trans fat is. It truly is a stealth fat. "One of the defining moments for me came when I looked at a box of breakfast bars," says Challem. "Half the fat was saturated fat, but there was no animal product in the ingredient list," he says. "This is in everything. It's like a wild card. It's as if you're screwing up how the body processes food."

The Labeling Battle

So the biggest problem with trans fat has been a simple one: No one knew how much of it was in our food. We eat only four kinds of fatty acids. Saturated, trans, polyunsaturated, and monounsaturated. The nutrition

A Dietary Fat Primer

Our diets contain only four kinds of fatty acids—monounsaturated, polyunsaturated, saturated, and trans. The first three are naturally occurring and show up in various amounts in everything from pork to flaxseeds. Each has a distinct chemical structure and works differently in the body. The body needs fats in the right proportion: Too much saturated fat, for example, can lead to heart disease. Too much polyunsaturated fat, which makes up most of the vegetable and canola oil we eat, can throw our overall fatty acid profile out of balance and keep our bodies from working their best. But the only artificial fat among the four—trans fat—is the one fat that the body doesn't need at all.

The fat we eat is never purely one kind or another. Butter, for example, is 63 percent saturated fat, with the remainder mostly monounsaturated fat. Olive oil is about 74 percent monounsaturated fat. Safflower oil, popular for salad dressings because it doesn't solidify when chilled, is about 74 percent polyunsaturated fat.

Within these naturally occurring fats are essential fatty acids, which are amazing workhorses in the body. They help keep cancer cells from forming, make blood clot, and help our brains work, among a host of other functions. The two essential fatty acids most of us know are omega-3s and omega-6s, and they sort of balance themselves out in the body. Too much of either can change the chemical and hormonal balances that make our bodies work.

Omega-3 and omega-6 appear in various levels in different foods. Fatty fish has a ton of omega-3s. Most Americans eat a lot of soy and other forms of polyunsaturated vegetable oils, and so they get too many omega-6s, which prevent the body from absorbing omega-3s. That's why largely monounsaturated olive oil seems to be such a healthy choice. With fats, it's all about balance.

labels on food must show total fat content, and then break out how much of that total is saturated fat. The FDA limits the amount of saturated fat in foods that make a "no-cholesterol" or "low-cholesterol" claim. But it sets no limit on trans fat. If the product makes certain health claims or if a manufacturer chooses, the poly and mono levels will be listed, too.

But until 2006, manufacturers won't have to specifically mention trans fat. (The exception is a handful of new products that proclaim they are trans fat–free.) But if there is trans fat in the food, those grams either get lumped into the total fat line on the label or show up in the monos and polys, which makes the fat ratio look healthier than it is. And because trans fat flies under the radar, food labeled "low in saturated fat," "cholesterol free," or "made with 100 percent vegetable oil" can have so much trans fat that those concerned about the health of their hearts would never buy it—if they knew.

After almost a decade of pressure from food and health advocates like Margo Wootan of CSPI, the federal government in 1999 proposed a final rule to force food manufacturers to add trans fat amounts to the nutrition labels on food packaging. But it has been a tough fight, and anti–trans fat advocates spent years battling tough lobbying from groups like the Grocery Manufacturers of America and the Food Processors' Association. The advocates' big break came in 2002, when the federal government agreed with what researchers had long been arguing: that there is likely no safe level of trans fat and that people should eat as little of it as possible. A study by the Institute of Medicine—part of the National Academy of Sciences and the medical body whose work is most widely used to set government food policies—confirmed that trans fat is directly associated with heart disease and increases in LDL cholesterol, the kind that can clog arteries. Consequently, the institute declared there is no safe amount of trans fat in the diet. But because trans fat occurs in so many types of food including dairy and meat, the study said an all-out ban would mean such extraordinary dietary changes that people might not get enough protein or nutrients. Instead, the government scientists declared that trans fat should be "as low as possible while consuming a nutritionally adequate diet."

Subsequently, the Institute decided not to list an upper limit for trans fat amounts in the diet—a first for any nutrient in food. It's that limit that the FDA uses to establish the recommended daily value for any part of the diet. That means the FDA will require food producers to list the grams of trans fat on the label with other nutrition facts, but it will not include the percent of daily value. There will be a note, however, saying that intake should be "as low as possible."

The fight for new labels has been a difficult one, in part because adding trans fat will be the first change to the national nutrition labeling laws since they became mandatory in 1993. And this change will be costly for manufacturers—not only because they have to rework their systems for breaking down the nutritional information on labels but because we might choose not to buy their products if we know how much trans fat is in them. But the change will cause consumers to save money on medical bills. The FDA estimates that Americans could save up to $1.8 billion in annual health care costs by reducing the amount of trans fat they eat. Many European countries are way ahead of the United States on the trans issue. In early 2003, officials in Denmark actually put a cap on how much trans fat could be in food. Only 2 out of every 100 grams of fat used in processed food can be trans fat.

Finally, in July 2003, the FDA made trans fat labeling the law. It's been almost a decade since the agency was asked to write a rule, and three years since it agreed to it. But food manufacturers still have until 2006 to comply. In the meantime, consumers are on their own. That's why it pays to be armed with some insider tips on how to avoid trans fat when you head to the supermarket or even your own kitchen.

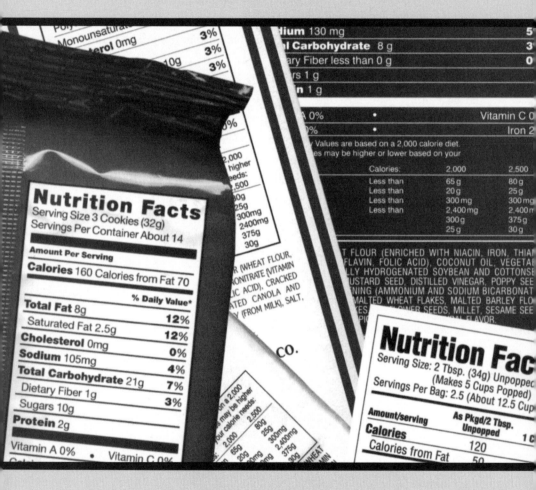

Po]y...
Monounsaturat...
...erol 0mg   3%
10g   3%
                                     3%

...0%

...2,000
...higher
...eeds:
...500
...0g
...25g
...300mg
...2400mg
...375g
...30g

Nutrition Facts
Serving Size 3 Cookies (32g)
Servings Per Container About 14

Amount Per Serving

Calories 160 Calories from Fat 70

	% Daily Value*
Total Fat 8g	**12%**
Saturated Fat 2.5g	**12%**
Cholesterol 0mg	**0%**
Sodium 105mg	**4%**
Total Carbohydrate 21g	**7%**
Dietary Fiber 1g	**3%**
Sugars 10g	
Protein 2g	

Vitamin A 0%   •   Vitamin C 0%

...ium 130 mg   5...
...l **Carbohydrate** 8 g   3...
...ary Fiber less than 0 g   0...
...rs 1 g
...n 1 g

...A 0%   •   Vitamin C 0
...0%   •   Iron 2

...y Values are based on a 2,000 calorie diet.
...es may be higher or lower based on your

	Calories:	2,000	2,500
Less than		65 g	80 g
Less than		20 g	25 g
Less than		300 mg	300 mg
Less than		2,400 mg	2,400 m
		300 g	375 g
		25 g	30 g

...T FLOUR (ENRICHED WITH NIACIN, IRON, THIAM
...FLAVIN, FOLIC ACID), COCONUT OIL, VEGETA
...LLY HYDROGENATED SOYBEAN AND COTTONSE
...USTARD SEED, DISTILLED VINEGAR, POPPY SEE
...NING (AMMONIUM AND SODIUM BICARBONAT
...MALTED WHEAT FLAKES, MALTED BARLEY FLO
...ES... WER SEEDS, MILLET, SESAME SEE
...PIC... XXL FLAVOR.

R (WHEAT FLOUR,
...NONITRATE (VITAMIN
...LIC ACID), CRACKED
...ATED CANOLA AND
...Y (FROM MILK), SALT,

CO.

...on a 2,000
...may be higher
...our calorie needs:
...2,000   2,500
...65g   80g
...20g   25g
...0mg   300mg
...2,400mg
...375g
...30g
WHEAT
MIN

Nutrition Fac
Serving Size: 2 Tbsp. (34g) Unpopped
(Makes 5 Cups Popped)
Servings Per Bag: 2.5 (About 12.5 Cup

Amount/serving	**As Pkgd/2 Tbsp.** **Unpopped**	
Calories		1 C
Calories from Fat	120	
	50	

Cooking and Shopping to Avoid Trans Fat

Ferreting Out the Fat: How to Determine If Trans Fat Is in Your Food

Adding trans fat to the list of things you need to think about when you shop for groceries might seem exhausting or even intimidating. It's tough enough getting the shopping done in time to get home and make dinner without having to read every label and calculate fat grams. But take a deep breath, because there is some good news about trans fat: It's fairly easy to eliminate this stealth food additive from your diet once you know what to look for.

The simplest way to avoid trans fat is to start to eliminate most processed and fast food from your diet. Of course, few people have enough time and motivation to cook everything from scratch. In fact, if you told me you planned to eat only crackers you baked yourself and never eat another fast-food french fry, I'd advise you to get a life. Still, it's not so hard to live without mass-produced frozen potpies, microwave popcorn, or cakes slathered with supermarket-grade frosting. And food manufacturers are warming to trans fat alternatives. Already, stores like Whole Foods and virtually any store with a decent organic or health food section carry plenty of frozen entrées, crackers, and baked goods that don't rely on trans fat. And these products are becoming better tasting all the time as the market grows.

If you're serious about limiting trans fat, the key tool is reading the ingredient label and doing a little math with the nutrition information listed on the package. Remember, the term "trans fat" does not yet appear on many nutrition labels and won't be required for a few more years. Until it does, here are some simple ways to discern if the food you're about to buy was made with trans fat:

1. Read the ingredients list. Look for the words "partially hydro-genated vegetable oil," "vegetable shortening," or some variation on the words "shortening" or "partially hydrogenated." It's the "partially hydrogenated" part that's important, because that's the manufacturing process that creates trans fat.

2. Check the order. Manufacturers list ingredients in descending order of amount. So if the phrase "partially hydrogenated vegetable oil" is listed among the first few ingredients, the product has more trans fat than if the phrase is close to the end of the ingredient list. Even some sports drinks like Gatorade have a tiny amount to give the product a better texture—usually far less than half a gram per serving. That might be an acceptable level to you, given that even people with the healthiest diets can't avoid eating a few grams a day. Just keep in mind that none of it is good for you.

3. Remember portion size. When you are deciding whether or not the product has too much trans fat for you, be honest about how much of it you are likely to eat. For example, most microwave pop-corn on the market has about a gram or so of trans fat per serving. But what's a serving? A cup. Can you remember the last time you ate only a cup of popcorn?

4. Consider quality. Trans fat is popular with food manufacturers because it is cheaper than healthier, better-tasting whole fats like butter or olive oil. Trans fat also acts as a preservative, meaning mass-marketed products like coffee cakes or muffins can stay on the shelf longer. An Entenmann's crumb coffee cake tested by CSPI showed that one slice had 2^1/$_2$ grams of trans fat, plus the same amount of saturated fat. The company's All-Butter French Crumb Cake had no trans fat. (But, it had 5 grams of saturated fat per slice, which doesn't make it the healthiest choice for someone looking to limit overall fat consumption or, specifically, saturated fats.) The point is that higher-quality products are generally made with higher-quality fats, like butter, and have less trans fat.

Want to get more advanced?

5. Do the math. In products that have the words "partially hydrogenated oil" in the ingredients list, note the amount of total fat listed and compare it to the breakdown of specific fats on the label. (See "A Quick Guide to Estimating Trans Fat" on the next page.) If the sum of all the individually listed fats doesn't equal the amount of total fat, the difference is likely the trans fat. The tricky thing is that not all food must list all fats. Heart-clogging saturated fat is the only fat required by law to be listed individually on food labels. Food packages that make specific health claims—like "low cholesterol" or "reduced fat"— often list poly- or monounsaturated fats along with saturated fats. Because trans fat is technically polyunsaturated fat, it is sometimes included in that category. The trick is to look for "partially hydrogenated" on the label. If it's high up on the list, chances are the remaining fat grams are mostly trans fat. If "partially hydrogenated" is low on the list or isn't listed at all, the unnamed fat grams are likely to be non-trans polyunsaturated fat or the less common monounsaturated fat.

A shortcut: In many products where partially hydrogenated oil is listed among the top ingredients, particularly cookies and crackers, you can make a ballpark estimate of trans fat grams by simply doubling the saturated fat amount. Wheat Thins, for example, have 6 grams of total fat per serving. Only 3 grams are accounted for, listed as saturated fat. That leaves 3 grams unaccounted for, which is likely all trans fat. Of course, this isn't exact, but it can be useful as a rough guide.

About Eating Out

It might be easy to control what you bring into your home to eat, but eating at a restaurant is another issue. Trans fat is the grease of choice in the fast-food and family restaurant industry. Most fast-food and family-style chain restaurants cook fries, chicken, and other foods in partially

A Quick Guide to Estimating Trans Fat

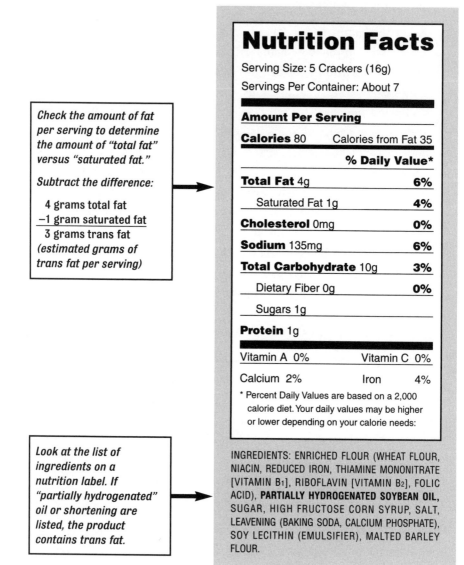

Check the amount of fat per serving to determine the amount of "total fat" versus "saturated fat."

Subtract the difference:

4 grams total fat
−1 gram saturated fat
3 grams trans fat
(estimated grams of trans fat per serving)

Nutrition Facts

Serving Size: 5 Crackers (16g)

Servings Per Container: About 7

Amount Per Serving

Calories 80　　　Calories from Fat 35

% Daily Value*

Total Fat 4g	**6%**
Saturated Fat 1g	**4%**
Cholesterol 0mg	**0%**
Sodium 135mg	**6%**
Total Carbohydrate 10g	**3%**
Dietary Fiber 0g	**0%**
Sugars 1g	
Protein 1g	

Vitamin A 0%　　　　Vitamin C 0%

Calcium 2%　　　　　Iron　 4%

* Percent Daily Values are based on a 2,000 calorie diet. Your daily values may be higher or lower depending on your calorie needs:

INGREDIENTS: ENRICHED FLOUR (WHEAT FLOUR, NIACIN, REDUCED IRON, THIAMINE MONONITRATE [VITAMIN B1], RIBOFLAVIN [VITAMIN B2], FOLIC ACID), **PARTIALLY HYDROGENATED SOYBEAN OIL,** SUGAR, HIGH FRUCTOSE CORN SYRUP, SALT, LEAVENING (BAKING SODA, CALCIUM PHOSPHATE), SOY LECITHIN (EMULSIFIER), MALTED BARLEY FLOUR.

Look at the list of ingredients on a nutrition label. If "partially hydrogenated" oil or shortening are listed, the product contains trans fat.

Nutrition Facts

Serving Size: 3 Cookies(34g)

Servings Per Container: About 4

Amount Per Serving

Calories 160   Calories from Fat 60

% Daily Value*

Total Fat 7g	**11%**
Saturated Fat 1.5g	**7%**
Polyunsaturated Fat 0.5g	
Monounsaturated Fat 2.5g	
Cholesterol 0mg	**0%**
Sodium 210mg	**9%**
Total Carbohydrate 10g	**8%**
Dietary Fiber 0g	**4%**
Sugars 1g	
Protein 1g	

Vitamin A 0%		Vitamin C 0%	
Calcium 2%		Iron 8%	

* Percent Daily Values are based on a 2,000
calorie diet. Your daily values may be higher
or lower depending on your calorie needs:

INGREDIENTS: SUGAR, ENRICHED FLOUR (WHEAT
FLOUR, NIACIN, REDUCED IRON, THIAMINE
MONONITRATE [VITAMIN B1], RIBOFLAVIN [VITAMIN
B2], FOLIC ACID), **PARTIALLY HYDROGENATED
SOYBEAN OIL**, COCOA (PROCESSED WITH ALKALI),
HIGH FRUCTOSE CORN SYRUP, CORNSTARCH,
BAKING SODA, SALT, SOY LECITHIN (EMULSIFIER),
VANILLIN – AN ARTIFICIAL FLAVOR, CHOCOLATE,
WHEY (FROM MILK).

*On nutrition labels where all
of the fats are listed, simply add
up the totals and then compare
this with the amount of total fat.*

1.5 grams saturated fat
0.5 gram polyunsaturated fat
+2.5 grams monounsaturated fat
4.5 grams

*Total fat is listed as 7 grams.
When you subtract the 4.5 grams
of other fats, you are left with 2.5
grams of trans fat per serving.*

hydrogenated oil, which often comes in a solid block and is then melted in the fryer. Cooks also slather margarine or another type of processed trans fat on griddles for pancakes and grilled sandwiches. Fish fillets, clam strips, chicken strips, and french fries all can have huge amounts of trans fat.

To get a sense of how much trans fat is in fast food, consider a Kentucky Fried Chicken Original Recipe chicken dinner. It has 7 grams of trans fat, mostly from the chicken and biscuit. Burger King's medium fries have 4.5 grams of trans fat. A typical fast-food meal has about 20 grams of trans fat. The CSPI tested onion rings and chicken fingers from family-style chains like T.G.I. Friday's and Denny's and found 6 to 10 grams of trans fat in an order. Even though some chains are using new liquid, non-trans oils for frying, some foods, like french fries, are sometimes par-fried in trans fat before they are shipped to the restaurants.

And you can always follow the advice of Harvard's Walter Willett (see page 9). In his 2003 interview with *EatingWell* magazine, he urged people to be persistent in finding out what fats restaurants use, and offered this example: "I was in West Virginia at a restaurant that had corn fritters, fried catfish, and fried green tomatoes on its menu. It sounded interesting. So I had the waiter go down into the basement and he got the label off the oil container that they were using for deep frying. And amazingly they were using non-hydrogenated soybean oil." Willett went on to enjoy every bite of those fritters and fish.

A Guide to a Trans Fat–Free Shopping Trip

The following is a breakdown by general food category, of products where plenty of trans fat is likely to be found.

BAKED GOODS

This is the heaviest trans fat territory. Generally, the higher quality the baked good, the less trans fat because more butter is used. Avoid

- Most mass-produced convenience and commercial bakery goods like cookies and cakes. Don't be fooled by innocent-looking cookies;

the majority of them, from vanilla wafers to animal crackers, have trans fat.

- Cakes and shortening-based frostings from supermarket bakeries.

- Cake and biscuit mixes are particular trouble spots.

- Doughnuts, which can contain shortening in the dough *and* be cooked in trans fat.

- Fried snacks, like potato chips and corn chips, have lots of trans fat. Frito-Lay sent samples of a new line of trans fat–free versions of Fritos and Chee-tos to newspaper food departments around the country, and they tasted much the same as the original products. The products have just gone into wide distribution.

- Crackers, particularly those with a "buttery" consistency like Ritz or Waverly, have lots of trans fat. But even relatively healthy-sounding crackers can have it. A box of reduced-fat Triscuits, for example, has 3 grams of fat per 7-cracker serving. Saturated fats make up $1/2$ gram and monounsaturated fats 1 gram. The crackers have no polyunsaturated fats, so the remaining $1^1/_2$ grams is trans fat.

- Croutons and salad toppings.

- Nondairy creamers and flavored coffees.

- Some premade dips, including some bean dips and spinach dips, rely on partially hydrogenated oil for texture.

- Whipped dessert toppings.

- Margarine. As a general rule, the softer the margarine, the less artery-clogging fat it contains. Margarine use is on the wane, and some statistics show it contributes less than a gram of trans fat to the daily diet of people who eat about 2,000 calories a day. There are some trans fat–free spreads on the market and increasingly these are labeled as such. Butter is still the best bet for flavor.

- Dry gravy and sauce mixes.

- Processed dinner aids like Hamburger Helper, Betty Crocker Complete Meals, or boxed potato dishes.

- Soup mixes.

- Refrigerator biscuits and piecrusts.

THE UNEXPECTEDS

These are foods you might not expect to contain trans fat. Avoid

- Some breakfast cereals. And note that even healthy-appearing versions can contain trans fat. General Mills Basic 4, which is labeled "low fat," has 3 grams per serving, 1 of which is trans fat.

- Breakfast bars. A Nutri-Grain bar has 3 gram of fat, but only $1/2$ gram is listed as saturated. Since no other fats are listed and partially hydrogenated oil is an ingredient, you can bet there's trans fat. Safeway Select's Healthy Advantage lowfat granola bars don't have saturated fat, but they do have $1/2$ gram of trans fat.

- Microwave popcorn, unless it uses palm oil, like Newman's Own Organics brand.

- Fish sticks or other breaded frozen foods. One sample of popular fish sticks had 3 grams of trans fat in a serving.

- Processed packaged puddings.

- Peanut butters that aren't made naturally.

- Frozen potpies. The Nutritional Action Health Letter showed that Pepperidge Farms Flaky Crust Pot Pie had 13 grams of trans fat. Marie Callender's Chicken Pot Pie had 16 grams of hidden trans fat.

- Frozen pizzas and other entrées, even if labeled as lower in fat.

- Frozen french fries and most other frozen potato products from the largest manufacturers, including Tater Tots. Some companies are exploring how to pre-fry their products in healthier oils, so make sure to check labels.

- Packaged instant noodles like ramen and soup cups. Look for packages where the noodles are steamed instead of fried.

- Some flour tortillas, although trans fat–free versions are available.

- Processed cheese, even those labeled lowfat.

- Powdered milk that is often added back into some brands of skim or lowfat milks. Check your milk label. Adding in powdered milk is a common practice at some dairies.

- Some food for babies. Graduates brand fruit and cereal bars, for example, have about $1/2$ gram of trans fat per serving.

How Much Fat Should You Eat?

The kind of fat and how much of it you need to eat depends on your size, how physically active you are, and if you are fighting a medical condition like heart disease. A very active man might need 3,600 calories a day, while a sedentary woman might need only 1,600. Here's a general guide:

For a person who eats 2,500 calories a day—that's what an active woman might need—about 30 percent or less of those calories should come from fat. That translates to about 80 grams a day, or 750 calories. Of that, only about 25 grams should be saturated fat, which comes from animal products like meat and butter. As a guide, keep in mind that a tablespoon of butter has about 16 grams of fat and 144 calories.

When it comes to trans fat, the Institute of Medicine has declared no level is safe to eat. But let's face it, totally eliminating trans fat from your diet is virtually impossible. Instead, consider this guide from the Alternate Healthy Eating Index, created by Harvard University researchers who conduct the largest study of eating habits in the country: The healthiest people, the researchers discovered, ate no more than 2 or 3 grams of trans fat a day. One glazed doughnut, which weighs in with 4 grams of trans fat, and you're over the limit.

Alternatives to Trans Fat in the Kitchen and Grocery Store

Although it seems like trans fat is lurking in every box and jar, food manufacturers are slowly starting to change fats and the formulas they use. "As the science has evolved related to trans fat, of course the industry is looking to different sources and re-engineering and reformulating products," says Bob Earl, senior director for nutrition policy and regulatory affairs for the National Food Processors Association. New, lower-fat margarines are being marketed as trans fat–free. Oil processors are mixing superhard, trans fat–free hydrogenated oils with liquid oil to make a suitable replacement. Cargill Foods sells a pourable, non-hydrogenated canola oil for frying, and for baking has a low-trans product called TransEnd that is only 2 percent trans. Nutritionists are revisiting tropical palm and coconut oils, which may not be as bad as once thought, and could actually have cancer-fighting properties. Healthier oils that remain stable at high temperatures are coming onto the market. The United Soybean Board, for example, is working with the USDA to develop soybean varieties that produce oils with a new kind of composition that makes the oils more stable so they don't need vigorous hydrogenation. Trans fat–free versions of canola and sunflower oils that can stay stable at high temperatures are coming onto the market, too.

Even McDonald's is working on a way to fill its fryers with oil that contains about half the trans fat of its current oil. It had pledged to cut trans fat by February 2003, but discovered the job was easier said than done. The company found that new, lower trans fat frying oils didn't deliver the taste of the former oil, and were much more expensive. But a representative of the company said McDonald's remains committed to finding a low trans fat formula.

As they did with organic produce and hormone-free meat, organic and natural food companies are leading the way to a trans fat revolution in food manufacturing. Peter Meehan, CEO of Newman's Own Organics, spent years casting around for a trans fat alternative so his company could produce Newman-O's, a takeoff on Oreo cookies. Meehan and his partner in the company, Nell Newman (yes, she's the daughter of Paul Newman and Joanne Woodward) finally found their answer in palm oil.

A Word about Coconut Oil and Shortening Alternatives

The search for a good alternative to shortening led us to two products, one of which we like a lot and another that just doesn't cut it.

The surprise in the kitchen is coconut butter, also sold as coconut oil. This is the same stuff that got such a bad rap in the 1980s, when a public campaign to stomp out heart disease made it a pariah (see page 6). True, coconut oil is one of the most saturated fats around—it's about 87 percent saturated (butter is about 63 percent, for comparison). One tablespoon has $12^1/_2$ grams of saturated fat. But here's the catch: it's a much different kind of saturated fat, one that is actually healthier than animal fat. And of course, it's healthier than trans fat.

Coconut oil is made up of medium-chain fatty acids that the body turns into energy quicker than other saturated fats. It has a huge amount of lauric acid, a great substance that is common in breast milk, has antiviral properties, can protect the liver, stop inflammation, and help metabolism.

For people looking for a shortening alternative, coconut oil stays solid at room temperature and behaves much the way Crisco does in the kitchen. When it's heated, there is a slight coconut aroma, but in baked goods like cookies, coconut oil provides a clean taste and a light, crisp texture. Mixed with butter, it gives a nice rise to cakes and pastry. Coconut oil lighten ups the richness of the butter a little, allowing spices and other flavorings to really come through. In baking, a ratio of a little more butter than coconut oil is about right. Coconut oil also works great as a medium for sautéing as well as for getting a crispy coat on fried chicken. It is more expensive than Crisco, for sure. But we think it is money well spent.

On the other end of the shortening alternative spectrum are palm oil–based products, which are showing up in the grocery store labeled as trans fat–free shortening. The versions we tried simply weren't worth it. They have a compact texture that is almost more crumbly than creamy, and an off smell that's vaguely industrial. In baking, the trans fat–free shortening makes for a denser cookie with an unpleasant texture. We suspect the disappointing results have something to do with how these new palm shortenings are processed. In some cases, palm oil can be a good alternative, especially for commercial applications.

A staple in many Southeast Asian kitchens, oil made from the fruit of the palm has almost half the saturated fat of regular palm kernel oil and is a breakthrough for baked products that used to require partially hydrogenated oils. Meehan now uses it in other cookies and in their microwave popcorn. Granted, a serving has 4$^1/_2$ grams of saturated fat, but it's much better than most microwave popcorns, which have 2 to 4 grams of trans fat in each serving.

For the kitchen, companies like Spectrum are producing palm oil–based shortening and cooking-grade coconut oil that behave the way traditional shortening does in the kitchen but are much healthier alternatives. (See sidebar page 25). Other snack and convenience foods continue to hit the shelves. Barbara's, a food company based in Petaluma, California, that makes cereals, cookies, and crackers, uses expeller pressed, high-oleic oils. And unlike a generation of health food products before them, these products actually taste better than what many of us grew up on. Try a box of their organic Go Go Grahams and you'll see. Amy's, another Northern California company, is doing much the same thing, as one of their trans fat–free potpies will prove. It easily beats out a standard Banquet potpie with 7$^1/_2$ grams of trans fat. Earth's Best offers organic teething biscuits made with canola oil. Even Legal Sea Foods, a respected East Coast chain of seafood restaurants, has figured out that taste, price, and health can come together. They've banned trans fat from their deep fryers and they even produce their own line of packaged oyster crackers that uses palm-based shortening. The little crackers are every bit as crunchy and crisp as any cracker with partially hydrogenated oil.

Figuring out who the good guys are isn't so difficult. Sometimes, it's as simple as where you shop. I spent an afternoon in a Whole Foods market in Northern California looking for trans fat. I read the labels on every packaged food I suspected might contain it, and never found the words "partially hydrogenated" on a label. And if you don't happen to have access to stores dedicated to eliminating trans fat, you can always read the labels.

Look for words like "cold pressed" or "expeller pressed," which mean the oils in the food were processed with a method that doesn't rely on heat or chemicals to extract the oils. Olive oil, coconut oil, palm oil, or liquid oils such as canola are a safe bet—as long as they haven't been partially hydrogenated.

And as a last word, I offer this. If you don't see what you want at your store or you have a question about whether the food at the restaurants you frequent are made with trans fat, ask. It's likely the manager might not have a clue what you're talking about or the restaurant kitchen fryer is filled with trans fat. But armed with a little information, you'll be able to avoid the deadliest fat in the American diet.

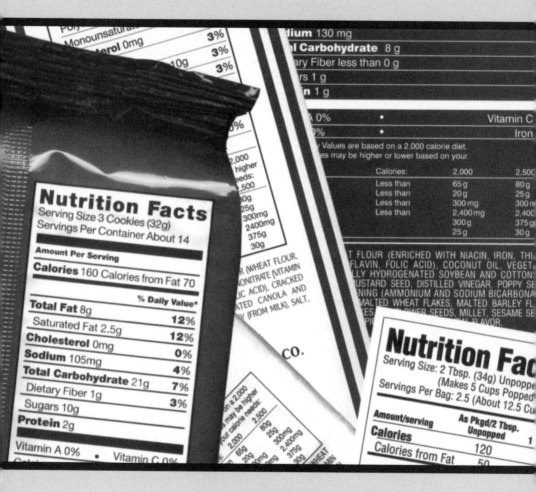

Poly...
Monounsaturat...
...terol 0mg   3%
...10g   3%
                     3%

Nutrition Facts
Serving Size 3 Cookies (32g)
Servings Per Container About 14

Amount Per Serving

Calories 160 Calories from Fat 70

% Daily Value*

Total Fat 8g   **12%**
  Saturated Fat 2.5g   **12%**
Cholesterol 0mg   **0%**
Sodium 105mg   **4%**
Total Carbohydrate 21g   **7%**
  Dietary Fiber 1g   **3%**
  Sugars 10g

Protein 2g

Vitamin A 0%   •   Vitamin C 0%

...dium 130 mg
...l Carbohydrate 8 g
...ary Fiber less than 0 g
...rs 1 g
...1 g

...A 0%   •   Vitamin C
...%   •   Iron

...y Values are based on a 2,000 calorie diet.
...es may be higher or lower based on your

Calories:	2,000	2,500
Less than	65g	80g
Less than	20g	25g
Less than	300 mg	300 m
Less than	2,400mg	2,400
	300 g	375g
	25g	30g

...T FLOUR (ENRICHED WITH NIACIN, IRON, THI...
...FLAVIN, FOLIC ACID), COCONUT OIL, VEGET...
...LY HYDROGENATED SOYBEAN AND COTTON...
...USTARD SEED, DISTILLED VINEGAR, POPPY SE...
...NING (AMMONIUM AND SODIUM BICARBONA...
...MALTED WHEAT FLAKES, MALTED BARLEY FL...
...ES ...OWER SEEDS, MILLET, SESAME SE...
... FLAVOR.

R (WHEAT FLOUR,
...ONITRATE (VITAMIN
...LIC ACID), CRACKED
...ATED CANOLA AND
...Y (FROM MILK), SALT,

CO.

...2,000
...higher
...eeds.
...,500
...80g
...25g
...300mg
...2400mg
...375g
...30g

Nutrition Fac...
Serving Size: 2 Tbsp. (34g) Unpoppe...
(Makes 5 Cups Popped...
Servings Per Bag: 2.5 (About 12.5 Cu...

Amount/serving	As Pkgd/2 Tbsp. Unpopped	
Calories	120	1
Calories from Fat	50	

...a 2,000
...may be higher
...calorie needs.
2,000   2,500
65g   80g
20g   25g
...mg   300mg
...00mg 2,400mg
375g   30g
...WHEAT

Trans Fat–Free Recipes for Your Favorite Foods

Notes from the Chef:
How These Recipes Were Born

In my career as a chef, I cooked for gourmets, celebrities, and other chefs. I sweated over dinners for three hundred and crafted appetizers with thirty ingredients. So when I had my baby daughter, naturally I planned to make all of her baby food. And, for a while, I did. I ground up organic brown rice to make her first hot cereal. I made carrot, fennel, and basil puree when she was ready for vegetables. I made mango and peach Popsicles when she started teething.

But, it seemed my little girl was not much of a baby gourmet. In fact, she preferred Cheerios, Eggo waffles, Ritz crackers, Pepperidge Farm Goldfish, and Wonder Bread. Well, I thought, at least she's eating something . . . maybe I could introduce the healthy foods later. I knew these foods weren't all that good for her, but how bad could they be?

Pretty darn bad, as it turned out. After reading my friend Kim Severson's articles about the trans fatty acids found in processed foods, I became concerned about the amount of trans fat that I might be feeding my child. I did a little research of my own and discovered that the scientists said that trans fat was even more harmful to children than adults. I looked at the nutritional label of the frozen waffles that my daughter ate, topped with Jif peanut butter, and calculated that she was eating double digit amounts of trans fat every morning. That was the day I vowed to eliminate foods containing trans fats from our diet. Since my little doll obviously had a taste for processed foods, I couldn't just start serving up brown rice and tofu—and who wants to eat like that all the time, anyway? My plan was to make healthy versions of the foods that she had learned to love.

I began with the waffles. After a few tries, I had an easy waffle recipe that froze nicely and could be warmed in the toaster with no loss of flavor or texture. I included flaxseed and wheat germ for extra nutrition, which also added a nice nutty flavor.

Then I started rooting through my cupboards (and my freezer) for other foods that I could refashion to eliminate the trans fat. I was horrified to discover just how many packages of food I had that contained hydrogenated oil, partially hydrogenated oil, or vegetable shortening. Around that time, Kim and I began talking about creating a book that would help other people to identify the sources of trans fat in their diet and to create alternative recipes for those foods.

Now, I am not a health food nut. Far from it, actually. And although I do have culinary training and have worked as a chef, I no longer have time to spend all day in the kitchen making dinner. I'm too busy working, playing with my toddler, and trying to find a little time to spend with my spouse. I like the convenience of packaged mixes and toaster waffles as much as everyone else. I wanted these recipes to be manageable for a weeknight dinner or weekend breakfast.

I began looking at ways to use other fats—coconut oil, palm oil, canola oil, lard, and, my favorite, butter—instead of vegetable shortening. When I tested the Spicy Buttermilk Fried Chicken recipe (page 70), I tried canola oil, peanut oil, lard, and coconut oil. Interestingly, the two solid-at-room-temperature fats (lard and coconut oil) fried golden brown and crispy chicken, while both of the oils (canola and peanut) made chicken that was blackened and greasy. Coconut oil became a favorite ingredient for crackers, biscuits, and piecrust, lending crispness and a flaky texture. I liked the clean, neutral qualities of canola oil for quick breads, pancakes, and cereal. Butter was a must for cakes and cookies, contributing rich flavor and light texture. Even lard found a place in my repertoire, making a very forgiving yet flaky piecrust perfect for meat potpies.

My little girl happily sampled her way through almost every recipe in this book. Her switch to a trans fat–free diet was easy and enjoyable. Now, she'll happily crunch a teething biscuit full of oat bran and soy protein, and her morning waffles are more wholesome. But the best part is that I know she's not eating them for the nutritional value—she's eating them because they taste good to her. That's a review that would please any chef.

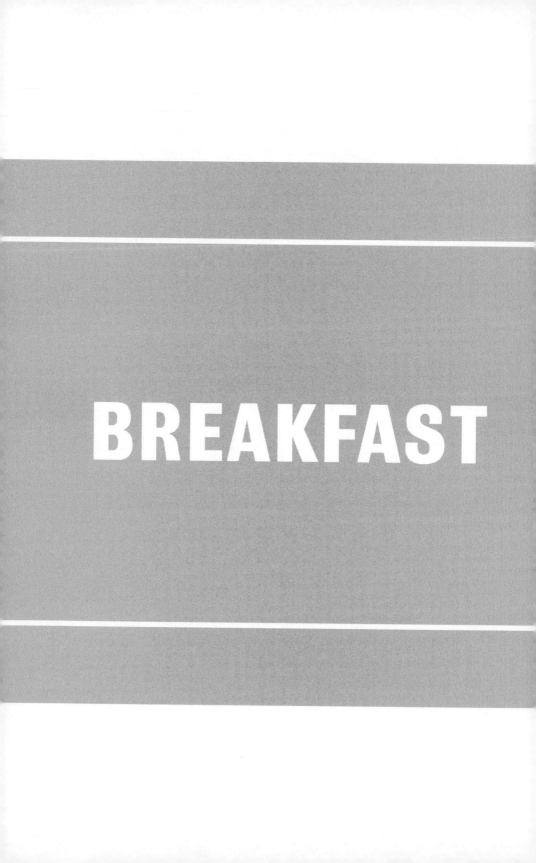

BREAKFAST

Maple Crunch Granola

MAKES 10 CUPS This granola is spiced only with a kiss of cinnamon to allow the maple syrup flavor to shine through. The rice cakes and puffed millet or rice add lightness and texture, and the whole grains and pumpkin seeds become brown and toasty in the oven. All together, these ingredients make a very satisfying, not-too-sweet, crunchy cereal. I buy millet and spelt flakes in the baking aisle (right next to the cornmeal) of my local supermarket. You could also try to find these ingredients in health food stores, the bulk-foods aisle, or online. I pair this granola with ice-cold milk and sliced bananas, or with a bowl of summer berries and vanilla yogurt.

3 cups rolled oats

1 cup spelt flakes

4 rice cakes, crumbled

1 cup puffed millet or puffed rice

1 cup sliced almonds

1 cup hulled pumpkin seeds

3/4 cup canola oil

3/4 cup maple syrup

2 tablespoons brown sugar

1/2 teaspoon cinnamon

1 teaspoon salt

1 cup chopped dried sour cherries or raisins

Preheat the oven to 325°F.

In a large bowl, stir together the oats, spelt, rice cakes, millet, almonds, and pumpkin seeds. In a small bowl, whisk together the oil, syrup, brown sugar, cinnamon, and salt. Add the syrup mixture to the dry ingredients, and stir to blend.

Divide the mixture between two large baking sheets, spreading it in an even layer. Bake the granola for 20 minutes. Stir and bake for 15 minutes more, or until lightly browned. Cool for 20 minutes, then stir in the cherries.

Granola can be stored for up to one month in a cool, dry cupboard. For longer storage, place 5 cups of granola in a freezer bag. Freeze for up to 1 year. Thaw before eating or you may break a tooth on the frozen dried cherries!

Cinnamon-Nut Muesli

MAKES 7 CUPS DRY CEREAL Muesli is a healthy whole-grain breakfast with no cooking required. I like this blend—the cinnamon mellows overnight, and the raisins and nuts soften, making a very creamy cereal. If you like hot cereal, warm it slightly in the microwave. Sliced bananas or peaches are the perfect complement.

Preheat the oven to 350°F.

Place the walnuts on a baking sheet in a single layer and toast for 10 to 15 minutes, until fragrant and lightly browned. Remove the baking sheet from the oven and allow the walnuts to cool. Chop the walnuts and set them aside.

Spread the wheat germ in a thin layer on a baking sheet and toast for 8 minutes, or until light brown. Remove the baking sheet from the oven and allow the wheat germ to cool.

In a large bowl, stir together the walnuts, wheat germ, oats, cinnamon, raisins, hazelnuts, brown sugar, and salt.

To serve, place 1 cup of cereal in a bowl and add $3/4$ cup milk. Repeat with 1 cup of cereal and $3/4$ cup milk per serving for the desired number of servings. Let the muesli soak in the refrigerator overnight. Serve warm or cold with fresh fruit.

1 cup walnuts

$1/4$ cup wheat germ

5 cups rolled oats

1 teaspoon cinnamon

$1/3$ cup raisins

$1/2$ cup hazelnuts, chopped

6 tablespoons brown sugar

$1/2$ teaspoon salt

$5 1/4$ cups lowfat milk

Quick Biscuits

MAKES 12 BISCUITS This is a classic biscuit recipe. I like using both all-purpose and cake flour, because the combination makes a fluffier biscuit. If you don't have cake flour in the cupboard, you can substitute 3/4 cup all-purpose flour for the cake flour (cake flour is lighter than all-purpose, which is why you use less all-purpose flour when substituting).

1 cup all-purpose flour

1 cup cake flour

1 teaspoon salt

2 teaspoons baking powder

1/2 teaspoon baking soda

6 tablespoons unsalted butter, cut into small pieces

3/4 cup buttermilk

2 tablespoons milk

Preheat the oven to 375°F.

In a medium bowl, combine the two flours, salt, baking powder, and baking soda. Using a pastry blender, your fingers, or a food processor fitted with a sharp blade, blend the dry ingredients together. Add the butter and blend until the mixture looks like cornmeal. Transfer the mixture to a bowl, add the buttermilk and milk, and mix it into the flour mixture with a fork.

On a lightly floured surface, pat the dough into a rectangle about 1/2 inch thick. Dip the rim of a 2-inch biscuit cutter or drinking glass in flour. Cut out the biscuits, dipping the cutter in flour before each biscuit. Gather together the scraps, flatten them, and cut the remaining dough into rounds. Arrange the biscuits on an ungreased baking sheet so the edges touch. Bake for 15 to 20 minutes, until the biscuits are light golden brown. Serve warm.

Any-Fruit-Will-Do Scones

MAKES 8 SCONES I always bake half of this mix at one time, and freeze the other half for another morning. These scones are not dry or crumbly like some; the addition of buttermilk makes a fine crumb with a light texture. I especially like them with fresh huckleberries, raspberries, or diced pears. Dried fruits, such as cherries, cranberries, or currants are also good choices.

Preheat the oven to 350°F.

In the bowl of a food processor fitted with a sharp blade, combine the flour, sugar, salt, baking soda, and cream of tartar. Add the butter and pulse 4 to 5 times in 10-second bursts, until the flour mixture and butter are blended to a sandy texture. Transfer the mixture to a large bowl and add the zest and desired fruit. Add the buttermilk and stir gently to mix the ingredients.

Divide the dough in half. Pat each piece of dough into a thick circle about 8 inches in diameter. Cut the circles into 4 equal wedges. Place the wedges on an ungreased baking sheet and bake for 35 minutes, or until golden. Cool slightly before serving.

SCONE MIX: Prepare this mix and freeze it for up to 3 months. After blending the dry ingredients and butter to a sandy texture, divide it into 2 equal portions (about 10 ounces each) and place them in plastic freezer bags. When you are ready to prepare the scones, preheat the oven to 350°F. Place 1 portion of the frozen scone mix in a medium bowl. Add 1 tablespoon orange zest and 1/4 cup dried fruit or 1/2 cup fresh or frozen fruit to the mix. Stir in 2/3 cup buttermilk. Follow the shaping and baking directions above.

3 1/4 cups all-purpose flour

1/4 cup sugar

1 teaspoon kosher salt

1 1/2 teaspoons baking soda

1 1/2 teaspoons cream of tartar

1/2 cup unsalted butter, cut into small pieces

1 tablespoon orange zest

1/2 cup dried fruit (such as currants, raisins, cherries, or cranberries), or 1 cup frozen fruit (such as blueberries or raspberries), or 1 cup diced fresh fruit (such as apples, pears, or peaches)

1 1/3 cups buttermilk

Cottage Pancakes

MAKES 16 PANCAKES Try a hot stack of these thin pancakes topped with fresh strawberries and maple syrup. You'll find they taste like a lighter version of a cheese blintz. I used to make them for my friend Sharon. She was a jogger, and the cottage cheese and eggs supplied plenty of protein for her after-brunch run.

1 cup all-purpose flour

1/2 teaspoon salt

2 tablespoons sugar

1 cup sour cream

1 cup small-curd cottage cheese

4 large eggs, beaten until foamy

2 tablespoons canola oil (for pancake griddle)

Heat a pancake griddle, a nonstick pan, or a well-seasoned cast-iron skillet over medium-high heat (about 350°F or until a few drops of water whiz around for several seconds before evaporating).

In a large bowl, stir together the flour, salt, and sugar. Add the sour cream, cottage cheese, and eggs and whisk until just combined.

Brush the griddle with canola oil using a pastry brush. Spoon a small circle of batter onto the griddle as a test. Adjust the temperature if the test pancake is cooking too fast or too slow. Ladle the batter onto the griddle, about 1/4 cup per pancake, but don't allow the pancakes to run together. Pancakes should be turned once and only once. Wait until the top of each pancake is covered with air bubbles (4 to 5 minutes) then sneak a quick look underneath. If the lifted edge reveals a golden brown color, the pancake is ready to flip. While you're waiting for the second side to brown (4 to 5 minutes more), resist the compulsion to press the pancakes down with the spatula. Flattening the pancakes does not cook them any faster and it makes your pancakes less fluffy.

Place the pancakes in a single layer on a baking sheet and keep them uncovered in a warm oven while you cook the rest of the batter. Serve warm with maple syrup.

Flax-Tahini Waffles

MAKES 16 WAFFLES Don't be frightened by these healthy-sounding breakfast treats. Even though they offer good nutrition and fiber, they are also delicious, light, and full of crisp, nutty flavor. If you don't have tahini, you can substitute almond butter or even good old-fashioned peanut butter. These waffles also make excellent toaster waffles, as described in the variation below.

In a large bowl, whisk together the two flours, wheat germ, baking powder, baking soda, salt, and flax. In a medium bowl, stir the butter and tahini together. Add the buttermilk, milk, sugar, and eggs to the tahini mixture and whisk until well-combined. Pour the liquid mixture into the flour mixture, and whisk until just combined.

Preheat the waffle iron. Brush the surfaces with canola oil.

Pour the batter over the waffle iron, covering about two-thirds of the surface area. Close the waffle iron and cook until the waffles stop steaming and are medium brown, 4 to 5 minutes. Remove the waffle and place it on a plate covered with a lid or an inverted bowl to keep it warm while you cook the rest of the waffles.

TOASTER WAFFLES: Following the instructions above, cook the waffles 2 to 3 minutes, until they are only light brown. Cool, then place in freezer bags. Waffles may be frozen for up to 6 months. When you are ready to use the waffles, reheat them in a toaster and serve warm.

1 1/4 cups all-purpose flour

1/2 cup whole wheat flour

1/4 cup wheat germ

1 1/2 teaspoons baking powder

1/2 teaspoon baking soda

1/2 teaspoon salt

1/4 cup flaxseed, ground fine

2 tablespoons unsalted butter, melted

3 tablespoons tahini paste

2 cups lowfat buttermilk

1/2 cup milk

3 tablespoons sugar

2 eggs, beaten

2 teaspoons canola oil (for waffle iron)

Raspberry-Almond Coffee Cake

MAKES 1 (10-INCH) ROUND CAKE OR 1 (9 BY 13-INCH) CAKE This coffee cake is easy enough to make on Sunday morning while your better half is still snoozing. It takes about 20 minutes to put this together and pop it in the oven. While it's baking, I relax with a pot of tea and the Sunday paper, and soon the house is filled with the smell of almonds toasting and cake baking.

2 cups all-purpose flour

3/4 cup sugar

1 teaspoon salt

1/2 cup unsalted butter, cut into small pieces and at room temperature

2 teaspoons baking powder

1/2 teaspoon baking soda

1/4 cup milk

1/2 cup plain yogurt

1 egg

1/2 teaspoon vanilla extract

1 teaspoon almond extract

1 cup fresh or frozen raspberries

1/2 cup sliced almonds

1/2 cup firmly packed light brown sugar

1 egg yolk

Preheat the oven to 350°F. Butter a 10-inch round springform pan or a 9 by 13-inch rectangular baking dish and lightly flour the pan, knocking out the excess flour.

In the bowl of a stand mixer fitted with a whisk attachment, combine the flour, sugar, and salt. Add the butter and whisk for 5 minutes, or until the mixture is finely textured with no large pieces. Remove 1 cup of the mixture from the bowl and set aside for the topping. Add the baking powder and baking soda to the mixing bowl and whisk until combined. Add the milk, yogurt, egg, vanilla, and almond extract and mix on medium-high for 2 minutes, scraping the sides twice. Turn the mixer to high and mix for 1 minute more. Fold in the raspberries with a spatula. Pour the mixture into the prepared pan in an even layer.

To make the topping: In a bowl, mix together the reserved crumb mixture, the sliced almonds, brown sugar, and egg yolk. Sprinkle the topping over the cake batter. Bake for 50 to 60 minutes, until a tester inserted into the middle comes out clean.

Cool for 30 minutes before serving.

Walnut-Cardamom Coffee Cake

MAKES 1 (10-INCH) BUNDT CAKE I just adore cardamom, and this indulgent coffee cake is perfumed with its spicy scent. Ground cardamom loses its pungency after a year or so, so use fresh spice for the best flavor. Serve thin slices of this sweet and rich coffee cake alongside a wedge of ripe cantaloupe.

Preheat the oven to 350°F. Butter and flour a large tube (Bundt) pan.

To make the batter: Using an electric mixer, cream together the butter and sugar in a bowl until fluffy. Add the eggs and beat to combine. Stir in the sour cream and vanilla. Fold in the flour, baking powder, salt, and cardamom.

To make the topping: Mix together the walnuts, cinnamon, cardamom, salt, brown sugar, flour, and butter in a small bowl.

To assemble: Pour half of the batter into the prepared pan. Sprinkle half of the streusel mixture over the batter. Cover with the remaining batter, and top with the rest of the streusel mixture. Bake for 1 hour, or until a knife inserted into the center of the cake comes out clean. Cool for at least 30 minutes before serving.

BATTER

3/4 cup unsalted butter

1 1/2 cups sugar

2 eggs

1 cup sour cream

1 teaspoon vanilla extract

2 cups all-purpose flour

1 teaspoon baking powder

1/2 teaspoon salt

2 teaspoons ground cardamom

STREUSEL

1 cup chopped walnuts, toasted (see page 35)

1 teaspoon cinnamon

1 teaspoon ground cardamom

1/8 teaspoon salt

1/2 cup brown sugar

1/4 cup all-purpose flour

1 tablespoon unsalted butter, melted

Cheese Blintzes

MAKES 8 BLINTZES Cheese blintzes are such a nice treat for weekend brunch. If you're pressed for time in the morning, make the crêpes the day before, wrap them tightly in plastic, and refrigerate overnight. Top the blintzes with sautéed apples, nutmeg, and brown sugar, or cherries simmered with orange marmalade and a squeeze of lemon.

CRÊPES

2 eggs

1/2 cup lowfat milk

1/2 cup buttermilk

1/2 cup all-purpose flour

1/4 cup whole wheat flour

2 tablespoons confectioners' sugar

1 tablespoon baking powder

1 tablespoon unsalted butter

FILLING

11/2 cups small-curd lowfat cottage cheese

1 egg yolk

1 teaspoon vanilla extract

2 tablespoons sugar

1/2 teaspoon cinnamon

1 tablespoon unsalted butter

To make the crêpes: In a medium bowl, whisk together the whole eggs, milk, and buttermilk. Add the two flours, the confectioners' sugar, and the baking powder and whisk to combine into a smooth batter.

In a small saucepan, melt the butter and set it aside. Heat a 5-inch skillet over medium heat. Brush the skillet with a thin coat of melted butter. Ladle 1/4 cup of batter into the hot skillet and quickly tilt the skillet to coat the surface with the batter. Cook for about 2 minutes, until the bottom is light brown and the edges of the crêpe appear slightly dry. Slide the crêpe onto a sheet of wax paper. Repeat with the remaining batter, brushing the skillet with melted butter before each crêpe and stacking the finished crêpes between sheets of wax paper.

To make the filling: In a small bowl, combine the cottage cheese, egg yolk, vanilla, sugar, and cinnamon.

To prepare the blintzes: Place 2 tablespoons of the filling in the center of each crêpe. Fold the edges toward the middle and tuck in the ends. In a large skillet, melt the butter over medium-high heat. Cook the blintzes, seam side down, for about 2 minutes, until golden. Gently turn the blintz and cook on the other side for 1 minute, or until lightly browned. Serve warm with the toppings of your choice.

Breakfast Burritos

SERVES 4 If you have leftovers from the Whole Wheat Flour Tortilla recipe (page 55), warm them up for these breakfast burritos. You can also find trans fat–free tortillas (made with canola oil instead of shortening) in most health food stores. The enchilada sauce, available at any grocery store, transforms ordinary eggs into a glowing orange scramble, and the chiles add a mild heat. I like my burritos simple, so these have only a few ingredients, but you can always pump them up with cooked chorizo sausage or cooked pinto beans. These make a great breakfast to go—just wrap them in foil to hold in the heat, and unwrap them as you eat.

In a large skillet, heat 3 tablespoons of the butter over medium-high heat. Add the potatoes and cook for 10 minutes, stirring occasionally, or until they begin to brown. Stir and cook for 5 more minutes, or until the potatoes are browned on all sides. Season with salt and pepper to taste and remove the potatoes from the pan.

In a medium bowl, whisk together the eggs, chiles, enchilada sauce, and green onions. Heat the remaining 1 tablespoon butter in the skillet over medium heat. Add the egg mixture and cook to a soft scramble, 3 to 4 minutes. Stir the potatoes into the eggs.

Place a tortilla in the center of a plate. Spoon 1/4 of the egg and potato mixture down the center of each tortilla and sprinkle with the grated cheese. Roll the edges of the burrito around the filling and turn the burrito seam side down on the plate. Repeat this process to make 3 more burritos. Serve with salsa and sour cream if desired.

4 tablespoons unsalted butter

1/2 cup cubed (1/2 inch) red potatoes

Salt

Black pepper

4 eggs

2 tablespoons canned minced green chiles

3 tablespoons prepared enchilada sauce

2 green onions, white and green parts, sliced

4 Whole Wheat Flour Tortillas (page 55)

1/2 cup grated Monterey Jack cheese

SNACKS & SIDES

Lemon-Pepper Crackers

MAKES ABOUT 16 (2-INCH) ROUND CRACKERS These light lemony crackers have a nice bite from the cracked pepper. Serve as an accompaniment to clam chowder or with any seafood soup. They are also tasty with herbed goat cheese and roasted red peppers.

$1/2$ cup all-purpose flour

2 tablespoons cold unsalted butter

$1/2$ teaspoon coarsely ground black pepper

1 teaspoon grated lemon zest

1 tablespoon sour cream

$1^1/2$ teaspoons freshly squeezed lemon juice

Kosher salt to sprinkle on crackers

In a medium bowl, blend the flour, butter, pepper, and lemon zest with a fork or your fingers, until well combined. The texture should resemble cornmeal. Add the sour cream and lemon juice and toss to combine. If the dough seems too crumbly, add 1 teaspoon of water to bring the dough together. Gather the dough into a ball, wrap it in plastic wrap, and chill for 30 minutes.

Preheat the oven to 375°F.

On a lightly floured surface, roll the dough out to a thickness of $1/8$ inch. Using a 2-inch round cookie cutter, cut out 16 rounds of dough. Place the rounds on an ungreased baking sheet, prick with a fork, and sprinkle with kosher salt. Bake for about 12 minutes, until golden brown. Transfer the crackers to wire racks to cool for 5 minutes. Store cooled crackers in a dry container for up to three days.

Pecan-Cornmeal Crackers

MAKES ABOUT 40 (2-INCH) ROUND CRACKERS   These nutty shortbreads fall somewhere between cookies and crackers—while the texture is similar to shortbread, the crackers are savory, not sweet. They are so good that they can stand alone, but they also make a nice accompaniment to a creamy blue cheese, such as Stilton or Cabrales. Toasting the pecans makes a world of difference in the flavor, so don't leave that step out.

Preheat the oven to 350°F.

Place the pecans on an ungreased baking sheet and bake for 5 to 10 minutes, until they are light brown and fragrant, but not too dark. Be sure to check them after 5 minutes; burnt nuts have a bitter taste. Remove the baking sheet from the oven and allow the nuts to cool. When cool, roughly chop the nuts and set aside.

Using an electric mixer, cream the butter in a large bowl until fluffy. Stir in the flour, cornmeal, sugar, and salt. Add the egg, mixing until well combined. Add the pecans, kneading them into the dough until evenly distributed. Gather the dough into a ball, wrap in plastic wrap, and chill for 1 hour.

Preheat the oven to 350°F.

On a lightly floured surface, roll the dough out to a thickness of $1/4$ inch. Cut the dough into rounds with a 2-inch round cookie cutter and place on an ungreased cookie sheet. Bake for 20 minutes, or until the crackers are light brown. Transfer the crackers to wire racks to cool for 5 minutes. Store cooled crackers in a dry container for up to three days.

$2/3$ **cup whole pecans**

$3/4$ **cup unsalted butter**

$1^1/2$ **cups all-purpose flour**

$1/2$ **cup yellow cornmeal**

1 tablespoon sugar

$3/4$ **teaspoon salt**

1 egg, beaten

Old-Fashioned Popcorn

MAKES 18 CUPS POPCORN Remember hearing that clink-clink-clink as the popcorn kernels hit the lid of your pan? No microwave popcorn can beat the taste of old-fashioned popcorn made on the stove. Peanut oil won't smoke at high heat, and it adds a nice toasty flavor.

1/4 cup peanut oil

1 1/3 cups popcorn

1 tablespoon kosher salt

2 tablespoons unsalted butter, melted

Heat a large heavy-bottom pot over medium-high heat. When the pot feels warm, add the oil, then add the popcorn. Cover the pot and listen for the popcorn to begin popping. When you hear it pop, reduce the heat to medium and occasionally shake the pan back and forth. When the sound slows to an occasional pop, remove the pot from the heat, carefully remove the lid, and transfer the popcorn to a large bowl. Gently toss with the salt and melted butter and serve.

Chewy Cherry-Almond Protein Bars

MAKES 12 BARS Bar none, these chewy protein-packed snacks are great for an afternoon nibble or to take along on a hike. Although they contain no sugar, the rice bran syrup (available in grocery stores and health food stores) lends a mild sweetness and keeps the bars moist and chewy. The optional chocolate chips make them completely irresistible.

Preheat the oven to 325°F.

In a large bowl, mix the puffed rice, bran, flour, protein powder, and salt. Stir in the coconut, cherries, chocolate chips, and almonds. In a small bowl, whisk the egg white, vanilla, coconut oil, and almond extract. Add the egg mixture and the rice bran syrup to the dry ingredients. Stir with a wooden spoon until the mixture comes together. Press the mixture into a lightly oiled 9 by 12-inch baking pan.

Bake for 25 minutes, or until light brown. Remove the pan from the oven and gently cut the mixture into 12 bars. Transfer the bars to a wire rack to cool for 20 minutes. Store the bars in a tightly covered container for up to 2 weeks.

1 cup puffed rice or millet

$1/2$ cup wheat bran

$1/2$ cup all-purpose flour

$3/4$ cup plain soy protein powder

1 teaspoon salt

1 cup sweetened shredded coconut

1 cup dried sour cherries

$1/2$ cup semisweet chocolate chips or carob chips (optional)

1 cup sliced almonds

1 egg white

$1/2$ teaspoon vanilla extract

3 tablespoons coconut oil, melted

1 teaspoon almond extract

$1/2$ cup rice bran syrup

Cheddar-Salami Cheese Straws

MAKES ABOUT 40 STRAWS   These cheesy sticks will disappear fast from any cocktail party or holiday celebration; the stripes of salami add spice and color. The process of making the straws sounds lengthy, but it's easy enough that a child can do it. In fact, it's not unlike rolling snakes of modeling clay and putting them together in a sheet of alternating stripes.

2 cups all-purpose flour

1 teaspoon salt

$1/4$ teaspoon dried thyme

1 pound grated sharp Cheddar cheese

$1/2$ cup unsalted butter, cut into small pieces

5 tablespoons cold water

3 ounces salami, cut into $1/4$-inch cubes

In the bowl of a food processor fitted with a sharp blade, blend the flour, salt, thyme, cheese, and butter until the mixture is combined well and no large pieces of butter remain. Transfer the mixture to a bowl, sprinkle the water over the top, and gather the mixture into a ball. Divide the dough into two equal pieces. Wrap one piece in plastic wrap and refrigerate; set the other piece aside.

Place the salami in the food processor and process until it is finely ground. Knead the salami into the reserved piece of dough, distributing the salami evenly throughout. Wrap the dough in plastic wrap and refrigerate for 30 minutes.

Remove the dough balls from the refrigerator and divide each piece into 6 equal parts. On a very lightly floured surface, roll each section into a rope about 9 inches long. On a large sheet of wax paper, arrange 6 of the dough ropes side by side, alternating the cheese and salami dough. Cover the dough with another large sheet of wax paper, and lightly roll them lengthwise into a 1/4-inch-thick rectangle. Place the sheet in the refrigerator to chill while you repeat the procedure with the remaining dough. Allow the sheets of dough to chill for 1 hour, or overnight.

Preheat the oven to 375°F. Spray a large baking sheet with cooking spray.

Cut each dough rectangle crosswise into 1/2-inch strips of alternating dough. Bake in batches for 10 minutes, or until golden. Transfer to wire racks to cool for 10 minutes. Serve warm.

Cheddar-Jalapeño Poppers

SERVES 4 Hooked on those hot and crispy jalapeño poppers? Me too! Instead of that oozy cream cheese, try this cheddar and cumin filling. These poppers are quite spicy-hot with a nice crunch from the fresh jalapeños. Canned whole jalapeños can be substituted if you can't take the heat. Needless to say, jalapeño poppers seem to require that you wash them down with an ice-cold beer or lots of iced tea.

16 whole fresh jalapeño chiles

1 cup grated Cheddar cheese

1/2 cup grated Monterey Jack cheese

1 tablespoon ground cumin

2 cups breadcrumbs

1 teaspoon salt

1 egg, beaten

1 1/2 cups buttermilk

2 cups peanut oil or lard

1 cup all-purpose flour

Slit the chiles down one side, leaving the stems attached. Using a teaspoon, scrape out the seeds and ribs. To reduce the heat of the chiles, bring a pot of water to a boil. Add the cleaned peppers to the boiling water for 2 minutes, drain, and rinse with cool water.

In a small bowl, toss the two cheeses with the cumin. Stuff each chile with the Cheddar mixture.

In a bowl, mix the breadcrumbs with the salt. In a shallow bowl, mix the egg and the buttermilk.

In a deep 9-inch skillet, heat the oil to 375°F.

Dip each chile into the egg mixture, dredge it in the flour, then dip it again in the egg mixture. Roll the chile in the breadcrumbs. Make sure to coat the chiles thoroughly with the breadcrumbs so the cheese does not ooze out into the oil as it melts. Repeat with the remaining chiles. Fry half of the chiles for 4 minutes, then turn and fry for 4 minutes more, or until both sides are evenly browned. Cool the poppers on paper towels while you fry the remaining breaded jalapeños. Cool for a few minutes before serving very warm.

Bistro French Fries

SERVES 4 TO 6 I used to make piles of these french fries when I began working at the Hunt Club in Seattle's Sorrento Hotel. Cooking the potatoes with peanut oil is the key—it makes very crisp fries. They are delicious plain, although some prefer them dipped in ketchup.

Cut each potato lengthwise into 4 thick slices. Cut each slice into strips; you should end up with 20 to 24 strips from each potato. Place the strips in a bowl of ice-cold water while you cut the remaining potatoes.

In a deep fryer or large deep pot, heat the peanut oil to 375°F.

Remove the potato strips from the water and drain them thoroughly on a plate covered with paper towels. If the potatoes are still wet when placed in the hot oil, the oil may splatter. Place the potatoes in the fryer basket and lower it into the hot oil. If you don't have a fryer basket, use a slotted spoon or spatula to carefully lower the potatoes into the oil. Cook for 4 to 8 minutes (depending on thickness), or until the fries are golden brown. Remove the fries from the oil and drain on a plate with dry paper towels. Add salt to taste and serve warm.

4 to 5 large Yukon gold or russet potatoes, peeled

4 cups peanut oil

Kosher salt

Flatbread

MAKES 8 TO 10 (7-INCH) ROUND FLATBREADS This dough is so versatile that you can vary the cooking method and make different kinds of flatbread. Bake the bread in a hot oven and watch it puff up to make a pita bread, or lightly grill it to resemble naan, the Indian version of flatbread. You can keep the dough refrigerated in a covered bowl for one week. The dough ages well, and will develop a nice sourdough tang after several days. When you want fresh flatbread, turn on the skillet, pinch off a lump of dough, roll it, and cook— you'll have fresh bread in five minutes.

1 package active dry yeast

1 cup warm water (110°F)

1 tablespoon honey

1/4 cup plain yogurt

1 1/2 cups all-purpose flour

1 cup whole wheat flour

1 teaspoon salt plus additional for sprinkling on top

1/4 cup olive oil, for brushing

In a large bowl, dissolve the yeast in the warm water, then stir in the honey. Stir in the yogurt. Add the two flours and the salt to the bowl and stir well with a wooden spoon. On a floured surface, knead the dough until it is firm and pliable, 4 to 5 minutes. Add additional flour if the dough is sticky. Return the dough to the bowl, cover it with plastic wrap, and refrigerate for 2 hours. (At this point the dough may be refrigerated for up to 1 week, punching it down whenever it rises to the top.)

When the dough has doubled in size, punch it down.

Preheat a 9-inch iron skillet over medium-high heat.

Pinch off a lump of dough about the size of a lemon, flatten it with your hand on a lightly floured surface, flip it over and flatten it again. Roll it into a 7-inch circle that is 1/4 inch thick. Brush the dough lightly on both sides with some of the olive oil.

Place the dough circle in the dry skillet. Sprinkle the top with salt. When the bread begins to puff slightly, at about 1 minute, flip it over. Cook until the bread is brown on the bottom, about 2 minutes. Flip it again and finish cooking the first side, about 2 minutes more. Serve the bread warm.

Whole Wheat Flour Tortillas

MAKES 8 TO 10 (8-INCH) TORTILLAS You'll be surprised how easy it is to make your own flour tortillas. While you can buy them at the grocery store, they often contain hydrogenated oil to maintain shelf stability. This recipe adds the extra nutrition of whole wheat, but you can also make it with only white flour.

In a large bowl, stir the two flours and the salt together. Add the oil and water and stir with a fork. If needed, add additional water to form the dough into a cohesive ball.

Divide the dough into 8 pieces, and roll each piece into a small ball. Cover the dough with a damp towel and let it rest for 30 minutes. On a lightly floured surface, roll each ball into 8-inch rounds. Stack the rounds between sheets of wax paper.

Heat a 9-inch cast-iron skillet over medium-high heat. Place a dough round in the skillet. Cook for about 2 minutes, or until the bottom is brown and the tortilla is slightly puffy. Turn the tortilla and cook the other side for about 1 minute, or until light brown. Repeat with the remaining rounds, wrapping the cooked tortillas in a towel to keep them warm. Tortillas are best served immediately, but can be stored, tightly wrapped in plastic, for 2 days.

1 cup all-purpose flour

1 cup whole wheat flour

1 teaspoon salt

2 tablespoons corn oil

2/3 cup water

Toasted Oat Tea Biscuits

MAKES 30 BISCUITS These little oat "biscuits" were created to satisfy my craving for the tea biscuits I was served at the Thistle Hotel in London. They are flipped like a pancake to make them crunchy, and make a wonderful accompaniment to a cup of tea.

2 cups rolled oats

3 tablespoons coconut oil, melted

1/2 cup all-purpose flour

1 teaspoon baking powder

1/2 teaspoon salt

1/2 teaspoon cinnamon

2 tablespoons unsalted butter, cut into small pieces

1/4 cup milk

2 tablespoons rice bran syrup or light corn syrup

2 tablespoons honey

1/4 cup brown sugar

Preheat the oven to 350°F.

In a bowl, toss the oatmeal and coconut oil together. Spread the mixture on a large baking sheet in an even layer. Toast the oatmeal mixture for 5 minutes, or until it turns light brown. Remove from the oven and cool for 10 minutes.

Transfer the oat mixture to a bowl. Add the flour, baking powder, salt, cinnamon, and butter, and mix until the butter is incorporated (the easiest way to do this is with your fingers). Add the milk, rice bran syrup, honey, and brown sugar. Stir until evenly moistened.

Drop the dough by teaspoonfuls onto an ungreased baking sheet. Bake for 10 minutes, or until golden brown. Flip the biscuits over and bake for 3 minutes more, or until the tops and bottoms are golden brown. Transfer to wire racks to cool completely. Repeat until all the biscuits are baked.

Whole Wheat Potato Rolls

MAKES 20 ROLLS A boiled, mashed potato is the secret ingredient that makes these whole wheat rolls light and airy—the starch in the potato keeps moisture in the dough while they bake. These rolls are wonderful hot from the oven. I always make them for Thanksgiving dinner, but they are too good to have only once a year.

In a saucepan, cover the potato with water and cook for about 35 minutes, until the potato is very soft. Drain, reserving 1 cup of the cooking liquid. Mash the potato with the reserved liquid and return it to the pan. Add the butter, sugar, and salt to the mashed potato. Allow the mixture to cool to 110°F (use a thermometer or hold your finger in the water for 10 seconds; it should feel warm but not hot enough to burn). Dissolve the yeast in the water and add it to the potato mixture. Add the eggs and stir well.

Transfer the potato mixture to a stand mixer fitted with a dough hook. Add the all-purpose flour and 2 cups of the wheat flour and mix for 1 minute. Add the remaining 2 cups wheat flour and mix for 3 minutes, or until the dough is firm and elastic. Cover the bowl with a towel and let the dough rise in a warm place until doubled in size, about 1 hour.

Punch down the dough. Tear off lumps of dough about the size of a golf ball, roll them into balls, and place on a large ungreased baking sheet. Cover with a damp towel.

Preheat the oven to 350°F.

When the rolls have doubled in size (30 to 45 minutes), bake them for 25 to 30 minutes, until light brown. Serve warm from the oven.

1 large baking potato, cut into 8 pieces

5 tablespoons unsalted butter

1/4 cup sugar

1 teaspoon salt

1 package active dry yeast

1/2 cup warm water (110°F)

2 eggs, lightly beaten

3 cups all-purpose flour

4 cups whole wheat flour

Roasted Red Pepper–Cheddar Corn Muffins

MAKES 12 MUFFINS When I worked as a chef, we served these as mini-muffins with an entrée salad of mixed greens, avocado, and spicy blackened salmon. The roasted peppers add color and complementary flavor to these cheesy corn muffins.

1¼ cups yellow cornmeal

½ cup all-purpose flour

1 tablespoon sugar

1½ teaspoons baking powder

1 teaspoon baking soda

1 teaspoon salt

1 cup grated Cheddar cheese

¾ cup buttermilk, at room temperature

1 large egg

¼ cup unsalted butter, melted

1 (7-ounce) jar roasted red peppers, rinsed and dried with paper towels

Preheat the oven to 375°F. Butter 12 muffin cups.

In a large bowl, whisk together the cornmeal, flour, sugar, baking powder, baking soda, salt, and cheese. In a small bowl, whisk the buttermilk, egg, and butter. Add the liquid ingredients to the dry ingredients and mix to just combine. Roughly chop the peppers and stir them into the batter. Fill the muffin cups half full with batter and bake for 25 minutes, or until a knife inserted in the middle comes out clean. Remove the muffins from the cups and cool on a wire rack for 30 minutes before serving.

Herbed Oven Fries

SERVES 4 TO 6 These chunky oven fries are sheer simplicity and are enhanced by using strong herbs such as rosemary and thyme. The key steps for crisp oven fries are using a heavy metal baking sheet, arranging the potatoes in one layer, and turning them only once during cooking.

Preheat the oven to 350°F.

Cut the potatoes lengthwise into 4 thick slices, then cut each slice into 3 pieces. Place the potatoes on a large baking sheet, toss them with the oil, and arrange them in a single layer. Sprinkle the potatoes with the herb, salt, and pepper. Bake for 35 minutes, then turn the fries with a spatula and bake for 30 minutes more, or until the fries are deep golden brown with a crispy exterior.

3 large russet or Yukon gold potatoes, peeled

2 tablespoons olive oil

1 tablespoon minced fresh rosemary, thyme, sage, or parsley

1 teaspoon salt

1/4 teaspoon black pepper

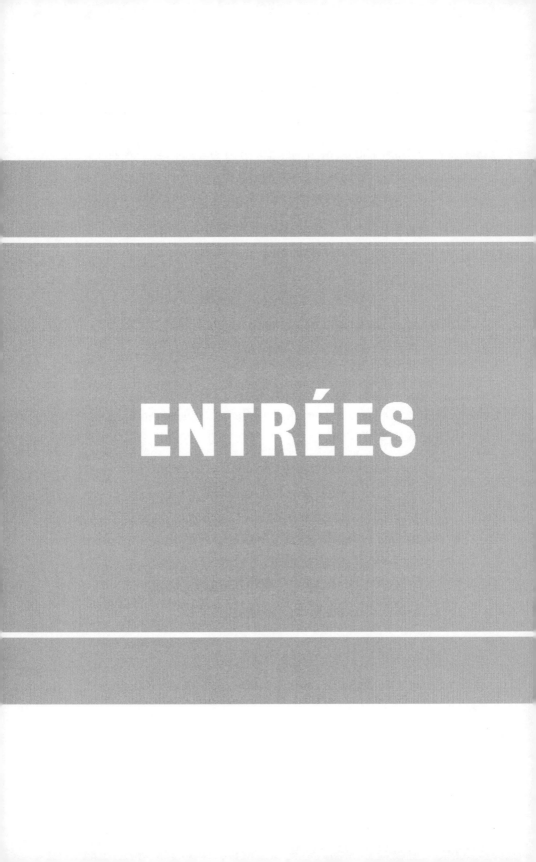

ENTRÉES

Beef–Shiitake Mushroom Potpie

MAKES 1 (9-INCH) POTPIE; SERVES 6 TO 8 Once you've had a potpie like this, you'll never want a frozen one again. With hearty chunks of steak, meaty shiitake mushrooms, and a savory gravy, this dish puts supermarket potpies to shame. The lard piecrust is sturdy, yet flaky, and works perfectly for this dish.

1 recipe Lard Piecrust (page 104)

2 tablespoons canola oil

1 pound beef sirloin tips, cubed

1/2 cup diced onion

3 medium carrots, sliced in thin rounds

2 tablespoons unsalted butter

1 cup sliced shiitake mushrooms

1 teaspoon kosher salt

1/4 teaspoon black pepper

1/4 teaspoon dried thyme

3 tablespoons all-purpose flour

1 ounce (about 1/4 cup) dried porcini mushrooms

2 1/4 cups low-sodium chicken broth

Prepare the piecrust dough and refrigerate according to the instructions on page 104.

In a large skillet, heat the oil over medium-high heat. Add the beef and let it brown on one side before turning it. When the beef has browned on both sides, remove it from the pan with a slotted spatula and place it in a large bowl. Leave the skillet on the stove.

Add the onion and carrots to the skillet and cook for 5 minutes. Add the butter, shiitake mushrooms, salt, pepper, and thyme. Sauté the vegetables for 3 minutes more. Stir in the flour and cook for 1 minute. Add the porcini mushrooms and chicken broth, and bring the mixture to a simmer. Remove the skillet from the heat, add the vegetable mixture to the beef, and allow it to cool.

Remove the disks of pie dough from the refrigerator, and on a lightly floured surface, roll 1 disk into an 11-inch round. Place the dough in the bottom of a 9-inch metal pie pan. Roll out the top crust.

Preheat the oven to 425°F.

Pour the filling into the piecrust. Wet the edges of the bottom crust with a damp pastry brush. Lay the top crust over the filling. Trim the crust to fit the pan and flute the edges. Cut 2 or 3 slits in the top of the crust to allow steam to escape while baking.

Bake the potpie for 10 minutes, reduce the heat to 350°F, and bake for 35 minutes more, or until hot and bubbly. Remove the potpie from the oven and cool on a wire rack to keep the bottom from becoming soggy. Cut into 8 wedges and serve hot.

Chicken-Tarragon Potpies

MAKES 8 (4-INCH) POTPIES; SERVES 8 Potpies are my favorite comfort food; they can be assembled from almost any combination of meat and vegetables you have on hand. Use this recipe for inspiration, but realize that potpies are very versatile. If you're out of carrots, increase the amount of peas. If you have an ear of corn rolling around your vegetable bin, toss the kernels in the mix. If you don't have enough chicken, substitute turkey or roast beef or use a rotisserie chicken from the grocery store. You can even make vegetarian potpies by substituting sliced button mushrooms for the chicken.

1 recipe Coconut Oil Piecrust (page 103) or Lard Piecrust (page 104)

3 tablespoons unsalted butter

1/2 cup diced onion

1/2 cup diced carrot

1/4 cup all-purpose flour

1/2 teaspoon salt

1/4 teaspoon black pepper

1/3 cup milk

2 cups low-sodium chicken broth

1/2 cup fresh or frozen peas

1 tablespoon chopped fresh tarragon

2 cups cooked chicken, diced

Prepare the piecrust dough according to the instructions on page 103 or 104 and refrigerate for 1 hour. On a lightly floured surface, roll 1 disk of dough into a 14-inch round. Using a knife, trim away the rounded edges to leave a 10-inch square. Cut the square evenly into four 5-inch squares. Place the dough squares on a baking sheet and chill them in the refrigerator while you repeat the above instructions with the second disk of dough.

In a large pot, melt 2 tablespoons of the butter over medium-high heat. Add the onion and carrot and sauté until the vegetables soften, about 3 minutes. Add the remaining tablespoon of butter and when it is melted, stir in the flour. Cook for 1 minute. Add the salt, pepper, milk, and chicken broth, stirring to combine. Bring the mixture to a simmer, then stir in the peas, tarragon, and diced chicken.

Preheat the oven to 350°F.

Place eight 4-inch ovenproof ramekins on a baking sheet. Divide the mixture equally among the ramekins. Top each ramekin with a 5-inch square of pastry and make slits in the top to allow steam to escape while baking (it's okay if the pastry hangs over the edges of the ramekin). Bake the potpies for 30 minutes, or until the crust is golden brown and the filling is bubbly and hot. Serve immediately.

FREEZER POTPIES: Prepare the pastry and filling as instructed above. After the potpie filling has cooled, top it with a pastry square, wrap it tightly with plastic wrap, and place it in the freezer. The potpies may also be frozen without the pastry topping, and topped with pastry or Quick Biscuits (page 36) dough just before baking.

To bake the frozen potpies: Preheat the oven to 350°F. Unwrap the potpies and place them on a baking sheet. Bake for 45 to 60 minutes, until the crust is golden brown and the filling is bubbly and hot. (You can also defrost the potpie in the microwave and then bake it for 30 minutes.)

Shrimp, Pepper Jack, and Feta Quesadillas

SERVES 4 TO 6 Quesadillas can be as simple as grilled cheese sandwiches, and they are just as easy to make. This recipe is a slightly dressed-up version of the basic cheese and salsa quesadilla. Use homemade tortillas or seek out a brand that uses canola oil instead of hydrogenated vegetable oil. You'll find these tortillas in the refrigerated section of the grocery store because, unlike the tortillas that contain shortening, tortillas made with canola oil cannot be held for weeks at room temperature. I like to use a creamy sheep's milk feta cheese for this recipe, such as a French or Israeli-style feta. The salsa makes more than enough for this recipe, so serve the extra with tortilla chips as an appetizer.

ONE-MINUTE SALSA

1 jalapeño pepper, seeded and stemmed

1 green pepper, cut into chunks

1/8 medium red onion or 1/4 cup sliced green onions (white and green parts)

1 basket cherry tomatoes

1 small handful cilantro leaves

Juice of 1 large lime

Salt

To make the salsa: In the bowl of a food processor fitted with a sharp blade, combine the jalapeño, green pepper, onion, tomatoes, cilantro, and lime juice and pulse 2 to 3 times. Add salt to taste.

To make the quesadillas: Heat a large griddle (or 2 large frying pans) over medium heat. Brush one side of a tortilla with oil and place it oil side down on the hot griddle. Spread a quarter of the pepper Jack in an even layer over the tortilla and top with a quarter of the shrimp and a quarter of the feta cheese. Drizzle 1 to 2 tablespoons of salsa over the toppings.

Brush another tortilla with oil and place it oil side up on the toppings. Press the quesadilla together lightly. When the bottom of the tortilla turns light brown (3 to 5 minutes), carefully flip it over with a large spatula and cook the other side.

Repeat the above steps to make 4 quesadillas, keeping the cooked quesadillas warm in an oven turned on low heat. Cut each quesadilla into 6 wedges. Serve with the salsa, and guacamole and sour cream if desired.

QUESADILLAS

8 Whole Wheat Flour Tortillas (page 55)

2 tablespoons canola oil

3/4 pound pepper Jack cheese, grated

8 ounces cooked bay shrimp (salad shrimp)

4 ounces feta cheese, crumbled

Guacamole (optional)

Sour cream (optional)

Southwestern Chicken Stew with Cheddar Spoonbread Crust

SERVES 6 TO 8   Think spicy shepherd's pie, and you have the concept for this moderately hot, hearty chicken and vegetable mélange. The spoonbread crust puffs dramatically like a soufflé when it comes out of the oven, so have your guests waiting expectantly at the dinner table so you can make a grand entrance.

STEW

3 tablespoons canola oil

3 boneless, skinless chicken breasts, diced

1 teaspoon salt

$1/4$ teaspoon black pepper

1 cup chopped onion

1 cup quartered button mushrooms

1 jalapeño pepper, minced

$1/8$ teaspoon cayenne pepper

2 teaspoons ground cumin

3 tablespoons all-purpose flour

1 cup diced tomato

3 cups low-sodium canned chicken broth

$1/4$ cup sliced green onions (white and green parts)

To make the stew: In a large Dutch oven or ovenproof skillet, heat 2 tablespoons of the oil over medium-high heat. Add the chicken, salt, and pepper and cook for 2 minutes. Add the onion and cook for 3 minutes more, or until the chicken just begins to brown. Add the remaining 1 tablespoon oil, along with the mushrooms, jalapeño, cayenne, and cumin and sauté the mixture for 2 to 3 minutes, until the mushrooms have softened. Sprinkle the flour over the mixture, and cook for 1 minute more. Add the tomatoes, chicken broth, and green onions and bring to a simmer, then remove the pan from the heat.

Preheat the oven to 375°F.

To make the spoonbread crust: In a large saucepan, heat the water over high heat. Add the salt. When the water boils, whisk in the cornmeal and cook for 30 seconds, whisking constantly. Remove from the heat and stir in the butter. Add the milk, egg yolks, and baking powder and stir well. Stir in the cayenne and cheese. In a separate bowl, whip the egg whites to stiff peaks. Fold the egg whites into the cornmeal mixture. Spread the spoonbread over the chicken mixture and bake until the spoonbread is puffy, golden brown, and cooked through, about 40 minutes. Serve immediately.

CRUST

3 cups water

2 teaspoons salt

1$^1/_2$ cups fine-grind yellow cornmeal

$^1/_4$ cup unsalted butter

1 cup milk

3 eggs, separated

1$^1/_2$ teaspoons baking powder

$^1/_8$ teaspoon cayenne pepper

$^1/_2$ cup grated Cheddar cheese

Spicy Buttermilk Fried Chicken

SERVES 4 TO 6 Fried chicken recipes always seem to call for frying in vegetable shortening, which is loaded with unhealthy trans fat. The coconut oil in this recipe has a neutral flavor, allowing the flavor of the chicken to shine through. The chicken is soaked in a spicy buttermilk marinade and refrigerated overnight to allow the flavors to develop. You could also marinate the chicken in the morning and fry it later that same day.

8 chicken thighs or drumsticks, or 1 whole frying chicken cut into 8 equal-sized pieces

2 cups buttermilk

2 teaspoons cayenne pepper

2 teaspoons salt

1 teaspoon black pepper

2 (14-ounce) cans coconut oil (4 cups)

2 1/2 cups all-purpose flour

2 teaspoons baking powder

1 teaspoon garlic salt

Rinse the chicken with cold water and pat dry with paper towels. Place the chicken in a shallow dish or bowl. In another bowl, whisk together the buttermilk, cayenne, salt, and pepper. Pour the buttermilk mixture over the chicken. Cover and refrigerate for 6 hours or overnight.

Remove the chicken from the refrigerator. In a large, deep straight-sided skillet, heat the oil to 375°F.

In a medium bowl, stir the flour, baking powder, and garlic salt together. Dredge each piece of chicken in the flour until it is coated on all sides. Carefully place the chicken in the oil; the pieces should not touch. Cover the chicken and cook for 20 to 30 minutes, until the internal temperature reaches 155°F. Remove the chicken from the pan and drain on paper towels. Discard the leftover oil. Serve immediately or refrigerate overnight for cold, picnic-style fried chicken.

FREEZER FRIED CHICKEN: The cooked chicken may be cooled, wrapped in plastic wrap, and frozen for up to 2 months. To reheat frozen chicken pieces, place them on a baking sheet and heat in a 350°F oven for 45 to 50 minutes.

Smoked Pork Chops with Potato Gratin

SERVES 4 You can stop buying those boxes of potatoes au gratin, which are loaded with trans fats, sodium, and mushy potatoes. This recipe couldn't be more simple—or more delicious. If you have a food processor, use it to slice the potatoes and you'll have a pile of even slices in a few seconds. Cream is the best choice for this dish because, unlike milk, it will not curdle during cooking. Smoked pork chops are sold already cooked, and should be warmed through rather than cooked again. When I take these potatoes out of the oven, I lay the chops on top and let them sit while I set the table. By mealtime, the chops are warmed through and ready to eat

Preheat the oven to 350°F.

Place the potatoes in a large bowl and sprinkle with the salt and pepper. In a 9-inch round baking dish, pour 2 tablespoons of the cream and then turn the pan to coat the bottom with the cream (this keeps the potatoes from sticking). Place a single layer of potatoes on top of the cream and sprinkle 2 tablespoons of the cheese over the top. Add another layer of potatoes and sprinkle with 2 more tablespoons of the cheese. Add one more layer of potatoes and pour the remaining cream over the top. Sprinkle the remaining cheese over the top.

Bake uncovered for 35 to 45 minutes, until the cheese is melted and the top is brown. Remove the pan from the oven, place the chops on top of the potatoes, cover with foil, and then cover with a dish towel. Allow the dish to rest in a warm spot for 15 to 20 minutes before serving.

2 pounds baking potatoes, peeled and cut into 1/8-inch-thick slices

1 teaspoon salt

1/2 teaspoon black pepper

1 half-pint whipping cream

2 ounces Parmesan cheese, grated (about 1/2 cup)

4 smoked pork chops

Curried Vegetable Empanadas with Cucumber Raita

MAKES ABOUT 36 EMPANADAS AND 2 CUPS RAITA   These golden pastry envelopes enclose a lively spiced-vegetable filling. You may want to make the pastry and filling one day and fill and bake the pastries the following day because the pastry has to chill for at least 3 hours or overnight. Use Madras curry paste instead of mild if you like spicy food. Patak's Lime Pickle is a wonderfully piquant Indian condiment that is often sold alongside Patak's brand curry pastes. You can leave it out, but it adds a unique flavor to these empanadas. I like them served with a cucumber raita, which is a cooling yogurt sauce that often accompanies spicy curries or other Indian dishes.

PASTRY

4 cups all-purpose flour

1 tablespoon salt

1 cup unsalted butter, cut into $^{1}/_{2}$-inch cubes

3 tablespoons mild Indian curry paste

1 egg, separated

6 tablespoons plus 2 tablespoons cold water

To make the pastry: In the bowl of a food processor fitted with a sharp blade, mix together the flour and salt. Add the butter and curry paste and process until the mixture has the texture of wet sand. In a small bowl, beat the egg yolk and the 6 tablespoons water together. With the food processor running, add the egg mixture to the flour. When the dough just comes together (about 20 seconds), remove it from the food processor and form it into 3 flat rectangles. Wrap them tightly in plastic wrap and refrigerate for 3 hours or overnight.

To make the raita: Heat a small skillet over medium heat. Add the mustard seeds and heat for 2 to 3 minutes, shaking the pan occasionally, until the seeds are warm and lightly toasted. Remove the seeds from the heat.

In a bowl, stir together the yogurt, cucumber, carrot, mustard seeds, lime juice, and cilantro. Add salt and cayenne to taste. Keep covered and refrigerated until ready to serve.

To make the filling: Heat a large skillet over medium heat. Add the oil, garlic, ginger, and curry paste and cook for 1 minute, or until fragrant. Add the onion, cumin, pepper, cloves, coriander, and cinnamon. Cook for about 5 minutes, until the onion has softened. Add the carrots and the cauliflower and cook for 5 minutes. Add the zucchini, pine nuts, raisins, and Lime Pickle and cook for 3 minutes more. Stir in the salt. Toss in the cilantro, stir, and remove the filling from the heat. Allow it to cool completely.

To assemble the empanandas: Preheat the oven to 375°F.

On a lightly floured surface, roll out one dough section to a 9 by 12-inch rectangle. Use a pizza cutter or butter knife to cut the rectangle into twelve 3-inch squares. Repeat with the other two dough sections.

Mix the egg white with 2 tablespoons of water. Place 1 to 2 tablespoons of the filling on each pastry square. Brush the edges of the pastry with the egg mixture. Fold the pastry over to form a triangle and use a fork to seal the edges.

Place the empanadas on ungreased baking sheets and bake for 10 to 12 minutes, until golden brown. Serve warm.

CUCUMBER RAITA

1 teaspoon mustard seeds

2 cups plain yogurt

1/2 cup peeled, seeded cucumber, grated

2 tablespoons grated carrot

3 tablepoons lime juice

1/4 cup cilantro leaves

1/2 teaspoon salt

1/8 teaspoon cayenne pepper

FILLING

3 tablespoons olive oil

2 tablespoons minced garlic

2 tablespoons minced ginger

2 tablespoons mild Indian curry paste

1 cup finely chopped onion

2 tablespoons cumin

1/2 teaspoon black pepper

1/4 teaspoon ground cloves

1/2 teaspoon ground coriander

1 teaspoon cinnamon

2 carrots diced

1 cup chopped cauliflower

1 medium zucchini, diced

3/4 cup toasted pine nuts

1/4 cup golden raisins

1/4 cup Patak's Lime Pickle

1 teaspoon salt

1/4 cup minced fresh cilantro

Roasted Summer Vegetable Lasagne

SERVES 8 TO 10 Make this tasty but easy lasagne at summer's end, when all of the vines and plants in your garden are loaded with an abundance of vegetables. Most garden vegetables can be substituted for my selections—try mushrooms, carrots, spinach, shelling beans, chard, or leeks. I mix the sauce in a large plastic pitcher and pour it over the noodles. Also, though you won't find this technique in any Italian cookbook, you can save yourself a dirty pot and some time by not cooking the noodles. Trust me, they will soften right up from the liquid in the tomato sauce and the roasted vegetables.

---

2 medium zucchini

1 red bell pepper, stemmed and seeded

1 small eggplant

1 medium onion, sliced

2 tablespoons olive oil

1 teaspoon salt

1 (16-ounce) container ricotta (or small-curd cottage cheese)

2 eggs

1/4 teaspoon nutmeg

1/2 cup Parmesan cheese

Preheat the oven to 350°F.

Slice the zucchini into 1/4-inch-thick rounds. Cut the bell pepper into 1-inch strips. Quarter the eggplant lengthwise and cut each piece into slices. In a large bowl, toss the zucchini, bell pepper, eggplant, and onion with the olive oil and salt. Place the vegetables on two large baking sheets and roast for 25 minutes, or until softened. Allow the vegetables to cool slightly before using.

In a medium bowl, stir together the ricotta, eggs, nutmeg, and Parmesan cheese until blended. In a large bowl or plastic pitcher, stir together the canned tomatoes, oregano, water, and sugar.

Pour 1¹/₂ cups of the tomato sauce into the bottom of a 9 by 13-inch glass baking dish. Place 3 uncooked lasagne noodles on top of the sauce. Cover the noodles with ¹/₂ cup of sauce, then top with a layer of roasted vegetables (about 3 cups). Place 3 to 4 slices of provolone cheese over the vegetables. Pour another ¹/₂ cup of sauce over the cheese. Top with 3 more uncooked lasagne noodles. Pour ¹/₂ cup of sauce over the noodles, then spread the ricotta mixture in an even layer. Top with 3 to 4 slices of provolone. Place 3 more uncooked lasagne noodles top. Spread the remaining roasted vegetables over the noodles. Pour the remaining 2 cups sauce over the vegetables and noodles. Top with 3 to 4 slices of provolone.

Cover the pan with foil and bake for 45 minutes, or until the filling bubbles. Allow the lasagne to cool for 10 minutes before serving.

2 (28-ounce) cans crushed tomatoes (or 5 cups tomato sauce)

1 teaspoon dried oregano

¹/₂ cup water

1 tablespoon sugar

1 pound lasagne noodles, uncooked

1 pound provolone cheese, sliced (9 to 12 slices)

Cornish Pasties with Caramelized Onions, Lamb, and Potato

MAKES 8 PASTIES A great way to use up leftover tidbits of roasted meat, these pastries were created in the tradition of those little meat turnovers popular in Europe and Australia. In Russia, they would be made with cabbage and ground beef; in Poland with turnips and pork sausage; and in England, they are often made with potatoes and beef or veal. These pies are versatile; you could easily substitute roast beef or pork for the lamb, as well as add other vegetables to the mixture such as peas, parsnips, or mushrooms.

1 recipe Coconut Oil Piecrust (page 103) or Lard Piecrust (page 104)

4 to 5 boiling potatoes (about 3/4 pound), peeled and quartered

3 tablespoons unsalted butter

2 cups thinly sliced sweet onions (Maui or Walla Walla)

1/2 cup sliced green onions (white and green parts)

1 tablespoon minced fresh ginger

1 tablespoon sugar

Prepare the piecrust dough and refrigerate according to the instructions on page 103 or 104. Place the potatoes in a pot, cover with water, and cook over medium-high heat until the potatoes are just cooked through the center, about 25 minutes. Drain the potatoes and set them aside to cool. When cool, cut the potatoes into 1-inch cubes and set aside.

In a large saucepan, melt the butter over medium heat. Add the sweet onions and green onions and cook for 25 minutes, stirring occasionally, or until the onions are soft and golden brown. Add the ginger and sugar and continue cooking for another 15 minutes, or until the onions are brown.

Add the chicken stock, marjoram, thyme, salt, and pepper to the onion mixture and stir to combine. Gently stir in the lamb and potatoes. Allow the mixture to cool.

Preheat the oven to 375°F.

Pinch off a lump of pastry dough the size of a lemon (about 4 ounces) and gently roll it into a ball with your hands. On a lightly floured surface, roll the dough into a circle about 7 to 8 inches in diameter and to a thickness of $1/8$ inch. Brush the edges with water. Place $1/4$ cup of the filling in the center of the circle, then fold the dough over it, forming a half circle. Beginning at one end, fold the corner over (like you would turn over the corner of a book page), and continue folding the edges of the dough in the same fashion, pressing the edges to seal the crust. Transfer to a large baking sheet. Repeat with the remaining dough and filling to make 8 pasties.

Bake the pasties for 25 to 35 minutes, until they turn light golden brown. Transfer to a wire rack, cool for 10 minutes, and serve warm. Leftover pasties can be refrigerated overnight and either served cold or reheated in the oven for 5 minutes.

$1/2$ cup chicken or beef stock

1 teaspoon chopped fresh marjoram

1 teaspoon chopped fresh thyme

1 teaspoon salt

$1/4$ teaspoon black pepper

1 cup roasted leg of lamb, diced small

ESPECIALLY FOR KIDS

Graham Crackers

MAKES 20 TO 30 CRACKERS Children love graham crackers, but unfortunately, they are full of hydrogenated vegetable shortening. This recipe has the flavor of graham crackers, and the coconut oil adds crispness. I use Bob's Red Mill Graham Flour, which is simply a coarsely ground wheat flour. If you can't find graham flour, increase the whole wheat flour to 1 cup.

$^1/_2$ **cup unsalted butter, at room temperature**

$^1/_4$ **cup coconut oil, at room temperature**

$^1/_2$ **cup sugar**

$^1/_2$ **cup whole wheat flour**

$^1/_2$ **cup graham flour**

$^3/_4$ **cup all-purpose flour**

$^1/_2$ **teaspoon cinnamon**

$^1/_2$ **teaspoon salt**

$^1/_4$ **teaspoon baking soda**

1 tablespoon molasses

3 tablespoons water

Using an electric mixer, beat together the butter and coconut oil in a large bowl for 2 minutes, or until well combined. Add the sugar and beat for 1 minute more. In another bowl, combine the flours, cinnamon, salt, and baking soda. Add the flour mixture, molasses, and water to the butter mixture. Beat for 30 seconds, or until just combined. Form the dough into a ball, wrap in plastic wrap, and chill for 1 hour or overnight.

Preheat the oven to 325°F.

Roll the dough between two sheets of wax paper to a thickness of $^1/_4$ inch. Cut the dough into 3 by 4-inch rectangles or use a cookie cutter to form the desired shape. Prick the dough with a fork. Bake for 10 minutes, or until light brown.

The graham crackers may be stored in a covered container for 1 to 2 weeks.

Teething Biscuits

MAKES 12 BISCUITS   I think of these cookies as baby biscotti, because they resemble those twice-baked hard cookies. Best for children over the age of one, these biscuits have just a hint of sweetness and a whole lot of nutrition. Cut them out with a round cookie cutter if you don't want edges to bother your teethers.

Preheat the oven to 325°F. Grease an 8-inch square pan with coconut oil.

In a medium bowl, stir together the oat bran, flour, salt, baking powder, cinnamon, protein powder, and dry milk. In a small bowl, whisk together the egg yolk, yogurt, rice bran syrup, and coconut oil. Add this mixture to the dry ingredients and stir to combine.

Oil your hands with a little coconut oil and press the dough into the prepared pan, smoothing the dough to make an even layer. Add 1 teaspoon of water to the egg white and beat lightly. Brush the top of the dough with the egg white. Bake for 40 minutes, or until golden brown. Remove the dough from the oven and slice it into 12 rectangles. Return to the oven and bake for 10 minutes more.

Remove the biscuits from the pan and cool them on a wire rack for 1 hour, or until completely cool. Store the biscuits in a dry, covered container at room temperature for up to 1 week.

$1/2$ **cup oat bran**

1 **cup all-purpose flour**

$1/4$ **teaspoon salt**

$1/2$ **teaspoon baking powder**

$1/2$ **teaspoon cinnamon**

3 **tablespoons plain soy protein powder**

2 **tablespoons nonfat dry milk**

1 **egg, separated**

$1/4$ **cup yogurt**

$1/4$ **cup rice bran syrup**

2 **tablespoons coconut oil, melted**

Fluffy Pancakes

MAKES 16 PANCAKES Pancakes are easy to make, but perfect pancakes need extra love and attention. If your fantasy pancake is thick but light, fluffy on the inside and golden brown on the outside, follow these instructions and you'll be a pancake pro.

2 cups all-purpose flour

1 teaspoon baking powder

$1/2$ teaspoon baking soda

$1/2$ teaspoon salt

$11/2$ cups buttermilk or 2 cups plain nonfat yogurt

$1/2$ cup milk

2 eggs

2 tablespoons unsalted butter, melted

Canola oil for cooking

In a large bowl, combine the flour, baking powder, baking soda, and salt. Place the buttermilk and milk in a large glass measuring cup and microwave for 1 minute, or until the temperature is 80 to 95°F. Whisk the eggs into the milk mixture until thoroughly combined. Add the milk mixture and the butter to the dry ingredients and stir just enough to moisten the dry ingredients. (Mixing more than necessary creates tough pancakes. Ideally, there should still be lumps in the batter.)

Heat a pancake griddle, a nonstick pan, or a well-seasoned cast-iron skillet over medium-high heat (about 350°F or until a few drops of water whiz around for several seconds before evaporating).

Brush the griddle with canola oil using a pastry brush. Spoon a small circle of batter onto the griddle as a test. Adjust the temperature if the test pancake is cooking too fast or too slow. Ladle the batter onto the griddle, about 1/4 cup per pancake, but don't allow the pancakes to run together. Pancakes should be turned once and only once. Wait until the top of each pancake is covered with air bubbles (4 to 5 minutes) then sneak a quick look underneath. If the lifted edge reveals a golden brown color, the pancake is ready to flip. While you're waiting for the second side to brown (4 to 5 minutes more), resist the compulsion to press the pancakes down with the spatula. Flattening the pancakes does not cook them any faster and it makes your pancakes less fluffy.

Place the pancakes in a single layer on a baking sheet and keep them uncovered in a warm oven while you cook the rest of the batter. Serve warm with lots of butter and maple syrup or fruit.

FREEZER PANCAKES: Prepare and cook the pancakes as instructed. Cool the pancakes on a large cookie sheet and then place the cookie sheet in the freezer for 30 minutes. Remove the frozen pancakes from the cookie sheet and place them in freezer bags. Label the bags with the date. (They taste best if eaten within 1 month, but they can be stored for up to 3 months with only a little decline in quality.)

To reheat freezer pancakes: Remove the pancakes from the freezer bag. Spread them with butter if desired, place them on a plate, and microwave on high for 60 seconds. Serve warm.

Homemade Peanut Butter

MAKES 4 CUPS The beauty of making your own peanut butter is that you can make it just as you like it. I like a little bit of brown sugar in my peanut butter, but you can leave it out if you prefer. This peanut butter also has a touch more salt than usual, which I find complements the jelly in a PB&J sandwich quite nicely.

1 pound unsalted peanuts

5 tablespoons canola oil

1¹/₂ teaspoons kosher salt

¹/₄ cup firmly packed brown sugar

Preheat the oven to 375°F.

Place the peanuts in a 9 by 13-inch baking dish and roast them in the oven for 8 minutes, or until light golden brown. Let the nuts cool for 5 minutes. In the bowl of a food processor fitted with a sharp blade, combine the peanuts, oil, salt, and brown sugar. Process until the peanuts are the consistency of peanut butter; this should take 2 to 3 minutes. If needed, add an additional tablespoon of oil to process the peanuts to a smooth consistency.

The peanut butter can be stored in a covered container in the refrigerator for up to 3 months.

Parmesan Chicken Strips

SERVES 4 TO 6 If your children love the chicken nuggets from the frozen food case at the grocery, have them try these chicken strips. They may not be dinosaur-shaped like the frozen nuggets, but they are tasty and almost as easy to prepare and they are trans fat–free.

Preheat the oven to 350°F. Cover a baking sheet with foil.

In a small bowl, toss the breadcrumbs with the butter. In a shallow dish, stir together the breadcrumbs, cheese, basil, and garlic salt.

If you are using chicken breasts, place them between two sheets of plastic wrap and lightly pound them to an even thickness. Cut the breasts into 1-inch strips. In a shallow dish, dip the tenders or strips into the milk, then dredge them in the crumb mixture. Lay the chicken on the baking sheet. Bake for 30 minutes, or until browned and cooked through. Serve hot.

1 cup breadcrumbs

2 tablespoons unsalted butter, melted

1/2 cup finely grated Parmesan cheese

1/2 teaspoon dried basil

1/8 teaspoon garlic salt

1 pound chicken tenders or 2 skinless, boneless chicken breasts

1/2 cup milk

Crispy Little Fish Sticks

MAKES 8 FISH STICKS; SERVES 4 I bought fish sticks for my toddler, thinking that I might get her to eat something "healthy" if it was covered in a crispy coating. I was horrified when I read the label and discovered that the coating was loaded with hydrogenated vegetable oil and trans fatty acids. Now, I make her these crispy fish sticks coated with oat bran, and she loves them.

1 cup lowfat buttermilk

1 egg, lightly beaten

1 cup oat bran

1/4 cup all-purpose flour

1/2 teaspoon salt

1 pound skinless, boneless fish fillet (halibut, salmon, or cod)

1/4 cup canola oil

In a shallow bowl, beat together the buttermilk and egg. In another shallow bowl (or on a plate), combine the oat bran, flour, and salt.

Cut the fish into 8 sticks. Dip the fish in the buttermilk mixture, then dredge it in the oat bran mixture, shaking off the excess coating.

Heat a large nonstick skillet over medium-high heat. Add the oil. Add the fish sticks and reduce the heat slightly. Cook for 4 to 5 minutes on each side, until brown and crispy. Drain the fish sticks on paper towels before serving.

Nacho Cheese Fries

SERVES 6 Most kids love nachos, and this recipe combines the traditional flavor of nachos with cumin-spiced oven fries. For adult palates, you can spice up the potatoes with 1/4 teaspoon of cayenne pepper before baking. Just like regular nachos, these fries taste great served with sour cream and salsa.

Preheat the oven to 350°F.

Peel the potatoes and cut each one lengthwise into 4 thick slices, then cut each slice into 3 pieces. Place the potatoes on a large baking sheet, toss them with the oil, and arrange them in a single layer. Sprinkle the potatoes with the cumin, garlic salt, and pepper.

Bake for 35 minutes, then turn the potatoes with a spatula and bake for 30 minutes more, or until the potatoes are golden brown with a crispy exterior.

Divide the fries equally among 6 plates and top them with the beans, tomatoes, cheese, and bacon.

3 large russet or Yukon gold baking potatoes

3 tablespoons olive oil

1 teaspoon cumin

1/2 teaspoon garlic salt

1/4 teaspoon black pepper

1/2 cup fat-free refried beans, warmed

1/4 cup diced tomatoes

1 cup grated Monterey Jack cheese

1/4 cup cooked and chopped turkey bacon

Mini-Pizzas

MAKES 4 (6-INCH) PIZZAS These crusty but tender pizzas can be on the table in just over an hour—with none of the trans fat found in frozen pizzas. Let the kids get creative with their pizza by letting them choose their own toppings. This is a great way to use up leftover bits of vegetables, lunchmeat, and cheeses.

2¹/₄ cups all-purpose flour

2 teaspoons salt

1 tablespoon honey or sugar

²/₃ cup warm water (100 to 110°F)

1 package instant (quick-rising) dry yeast

2 tablespoons olive oil

Pizza sauce (tomato, pesto, olive oil)

Cheese (mozzarella, provolone, gouda, parmesan, feta)

Pizza toppings (cherry tomatoes, fresh basil, red onion, green onions, mushrooms, peppers, fresh spinach, zucchini, olives, artichoke hearts, salad shrimp, ground beef, bacon, ham, sausage, smoked turkey, chicken)

Heat the oven to 200°F for 10 minutes and then turn it off.

In the bowl of a stand mixer fitted with a dough hook, combine the flour and salt. In a small bowl, stir the honey into the water, then add the yeast and stir to dissolve. Add the yeast mixture and the olive oil to the mixer bowl. Mix on low for 1 minute; increase the speed to medium and mix for 1 minute more.

Place the dough in a large bowl, cover it with plastic wrap, and place it in the warm oven for 30 minutes, or until the dough has nearly doubled in size. Punch the dough down, and divide it into 4 pieces. Place a dough piece on a lightly oiled pizza stone or baking sheet and use your fingers to gently press it out into a thin 6-inch round. Repeat with the remaining dough. (At this point, the dough can be frozen for up to 6 months if desired.)

Preheat the oven to 350°F.

Allow the pizza dough to rise for 15 minutes, then top each round with sauce, cheese, and toppings of your choice. Bake for 20 minutes, or until golden brown, and serve warm.

Apple Pocket Pies

MAKES 8 POCKET PIES Coconut Oil Piecrust (page 103) is the perfect pastry for these little apple pocket pies. They bake up puffy, flaky, and tender. I like to combine at least two varieties of apples, which adds a little complexity to the flavor. Kids can help with the assembly; have them spoon the apples into the center and pinch the edges of the crust together.

Prepare the piecrust dough and refrigerate according to the instructions on page 103.

Peel and the core apples, cut into 1-inch chunks, and toss with the lemon juice in a bowl. In a medium skillet, melt the coconut oil over low heat until it liquefies. Add the apples, brown sugar, and cinnamon and sauté for about 5 minutes, until the apples are softened. Return the apple mixture to the bowl while you prepare the pastry squares.

Preheat the oven to 400°F.

Divide the chilled pie dough into 2 portions. Roll each portion between 2 sheets of waxed paper into a 10-inch square. Remove the top sheet of waxed paper, trim the edges of the dough, and cut it into 4 equal squares. Spoon 2 heaping tablespoons of the apple mixture into the center of each square. Fold in half to form a triangle and seal the edges by pressing them together with the tines of a fork dipped in flour. Repeat with the remaining dough. Use the waxed paper sheet to transfer the pastries onto a large, nonstick baking sheet. Bake for 20 minutes, or until the crust is puffed and light brown. Cool on the baking sheet, then transfer the pastries to a plate with a spatula. Serve warm or at room temperature.

1 recipe Coconut Oil Piecrust (page 103)

5 apples, a mix of Granny Smith and Macintosh

2 teaspoons lemon juice

1 tablespoon coconut oil

1/4 cup firmly packed brown sugar

1/4 teaspoon cinnamon

Ice Cream Sandwiches

MAKES 8 ICE CREAM SANDWICHES I was shocked when I started reading the nutrition labels on ice cream sandwiches. They all seem to contain hydrogenated vegetable oils, and most have an abundance of artificial flavorings and ingredients. I decided to try making my own, and am very happy with the results. Because lowfat ice cream has a less creamy texture and melts very quickly, use a full-fat ice cream made with natural ingredients for this recipe.

2 cups all-purpose flour

$3/4$ cup Dutch-process cocoa

$1/2$ teaspoon cinnamon

Pinch of salt

1 cup unsalted butter, at room temperature

2 cups confectioners' sugar

1 whole egg plus 1 egg yolk

1 teaspoon vanilla extract

$1^1/2$ pints (3 cups) vanilla ice cream

1 cup finely chopped almonds (optional)

1 cup crushed toffee candy bars (optional)

1 cup miniature chocolate chips (optional)

To make the cookies: In a bowl, whisk together the flour, cocoa, cinnamon, and salt and set aside. In a large bowl and using an electric mixer, beat the butter until it is light and fluffy. Add the sugar and beat to combine. Add the egg, egg yolk, and vanilla, and beat for 1 minute, or until the mixture is thick and fluffy and has the appearance of frosting. Stir in the flour mixture until it is combined into a firm dough. Divide the dough in half. Form each half into a flat disk, wrap in plastic wrap , and refrigerate for 2 hours, or until firm.

Preheat the oven to 350°F.

On a lightly floured surface, roll each disk of dough to a thickness of $1/8$ inch. Using a 3-inch round cookie cutter, cut out the cookies. Gather together the scraps, flatten them, and cut the remaining dough into cookies. Place them on an ungreased baking sheet 1 inch apart. Bake for 10 minutes. The color will not change noticeably, but the cookies will appear baked and slightly puffed. Cool on the baking sheet for 5 minutes before transferring the cookies to a wire rack. Cool the cookies for 1 hour, or until completely cooled.

To assemble the ice cream sandwiches: Remove the ice cream from the freezer and allow it to sit at room temperature for 15 minutes. Place the almonds, toffee, and chocolate chips in three shallow dishes. Scoop $1/3$ cup ice cream onto a cookie, spreading it evenly to the edges with a spatula or spoon. Top the ice cream with another cookie and press down lightly. Roll the edges of the ice cream sandwich in the toppings as desired. Repeat to make 8 ice cream sandwiches. Serve immediately or place the sandwiches in freezer bags and freeze them for up to 4 weeks.

SANDWICH COOKIES: If ice cream sandwiches seem too decadent for your taste, this cookie recipe is delicious on its own.

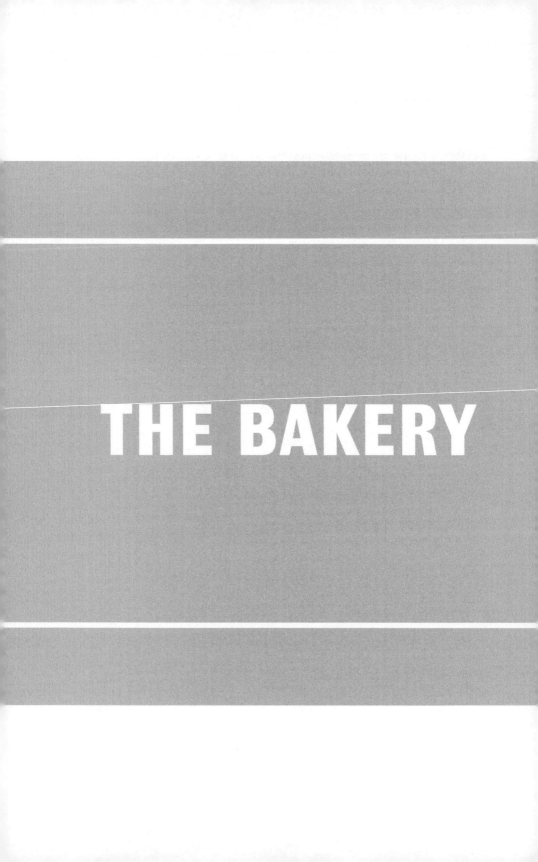

THE BAKERY

White Bread

MAKES 2 LOAVES If you read the labels on commercial bread, you'll find that nearly every loaf contains hydrogenated vegetable oils. If you eat as much bread as I do, you'll want to have an alternative to the bread at your grocery. This recipe makes one loaf for now and one loaf to freeze for later. For a softer crust, brush the tops with melted butter right after the loaves come out of the oven.

2 cups milk

1/4 cup unsalted butter, at room temperature

2 teaspoons salt

1/2 cup sugar

1/2 cup warm water (110°F)

1 package active dry yeast

6 to 7 cups bread flour

Grease two 9 by 5-inch loaf pans.

In a saucepan, heat the milk to a simmer over medium heat. Add the butter, salt, and 1/4 cup of the sugar. Remove the milk mixture from the heat and allow it to cool until just warm (about 110°F).

In a large bowl, place the water and the remaining 1/4 cup sugar. Sprinkle the yeast over the top and stir to blend. Add the milk mixture to the yeast. Stir 6 cups of the flour into the liquid. If needed, add the additional flour until you have a soft but firm dough. On a lightly floured surface, knead the dough until it is smooth and elastic (6 to 10 minutes). Place the dough in a lightly greased bowl, cover, and place it in a warm spot to rise.

When the dough has doubled in size, after about 11/2 hours, punch the dough down. Shape the dough into 2 loaves, place them in the prepared pans, cover, and let them rise again, until the loaves are about 1 inch above the sides of the pans, about 1 hour.

Preheat the oven to 350°F.

Bake the loaves for 30 to 40 minutes, until golden brown. Remove the loaves from the pans and cool the bread on a rack for 40 minutes before slicing.

Caraway-Raisin Soda Bread

MAKES 2 LOAVES Similar to an Irish soda bread, this loaf has a rustic appearance but sophisticated flavors. I like to serve this bread as an accompaniment to carrot or potato soups. It also makes a wickedly good grilled cheese sandwich when spread with a very thin layer of Dijon mustard and topped with a nutty cheese such as Comte or Gouda.

Preheat the oven to 375°F. Grease and flour two 9 by 5-inch loaf pans, shaking out the excess flour.

In a large bowl, whisk together the buttermilk, eggs, baking soda, honey, and cornmeal. In another large bowl, combine the two flours, salt, baking powder, caraway seeds, and the raisins. Pour the milk mixture into the flour mixture and stir well. Divide the batter equally between the two pans.

Bake the bread for about 75 minutes. Test for doneness by inserting a knife into the center of the loaf. If the knife comes out clean, remove the pans from the oven and cool the loaves in the pan for 15 minutes. Remove the loaves from the pan and cool completely before slicing.

4 cups buttermilk, at room temperature

2 eggs, lightly beaten

1/2 teaspoon baking soda

1/4 cup honey

1/3 cup yellow cornmeal

3 cups whole wheat flour

4 cups all-purpose flour

1 tablespoon salt

2 tablespoons plus 2 teaspoons baking powder

1/2 cup caraway seeds

2 cups raisins

Lemony Yogurt Muffins

MAKES 12 MUFFINS These muffins are just slightly sweet, and have light brown tops with a pebbly texture. About 20 years ago, I cut a recipe for lemon muffins out of the *Washington Post* and have fiddled with it ever since. The original recipe called for sour cream, but I prefer to use yogurt because it adds a tangy flavor that complements the lemon. Yogurt is also much lower in fat and calories than sour cream. Drenching the muffins with lemon syrup while they are still warm punches up the lemon flavor.

2 cups all-purpose flour

1/4 teaspoon salt

1 teaspoon baking powder

1 teaspoon baking soda

2 eggs

1 1/4 cups plain yogurt

1/4 cup sugar

1/2 cup unsalted butter, melted

1 tablespoon lemon zest

1/2 cup lemon juice

1/2 cup sugar

2 tablespoons water

Preheat the oven to 350°F. Spray a muffin tin with cooking spray.

In a small bowl, whisk together the flour, salt, baking powder, and baking soda. In a large bowl, whisk the eggs, yogurt, sugar, butter, and zest. Add the flour mixture, and whisk until just combined. Divide the batter among the muffin cups. Bake the muffins for 20 minutes, or until golden.

While the muffins are baking, make the syrup. In a saucepan, place the lemon juice, sugar, and water. Bring to a boil and cook for 1 minute. Remove from the heat and set aside.

When the muffins come out of the oven, pierce the tops with a fork. Pour the syrup over the muffins, letting it run inside the muffin cups. Cool for 10 minutes, then remove the muffins from the tin and finish cooling them on a wire rack.

Oatmeal-Chocolate-Cherry Cookies

MAKES 16 LARGE COOKIES The combination of cherries and chocolate brings these cookies to a level previously unknown in an oatmeal cookie. Making the cookies larger than a typical cookie keeps them chewy and tender. If you like smaller cookies, use a tablespoon to portion them, and bake for a minute or two less.

Preheat the oven to 350°F.

Using an electric mixer, beat the butter and two sugars in a large bowl until the mixture is light and fluffy. Add the eggs and vanilla and beat until smooth, about 1 minute. Stir in the flour, baking powder, and salt, mixing until well combined. Stir in the oats, cherries, and chocolate.

Using an ice-cream scoop, form a ball of dough the size of an egg. Flatten the ball slightly and place it on a large cookie sheet. Repeat with the remaining dough, spacing the cookies about 1 inch apart. Bake in two batches for 20 minutes, or until light brown. Remove the cookies from the baking sheet to cool on a wire rack.

1 cup unsalted butter, at room temperature

1 cup sugar

1 cup brown sugar

2 eggs

2 teaspoons vanilla extract

2 cups all-purpose flour

$1/2$ teaspoon baking powder

1 teaspoon salt

3 cups rolled oats

$1/2$ cup dried sour cherries

1 cup (about 6 ounces) chopped bittersweet chocolate

Chocolate Chip Cookies

MAKES ABOUT 48 COOKIES   I always liked the classic Toll House chocolate chip cookie recipe on the back of those yellow bags of semisweet chips, but I thought I could improve on it and make the cookies just a touch more nutritious. These cookies are puffed and tall, with plenty of chocolate chips.

1 cup unsalted butter, at room temperature

1/2 cup sugar

1 cup brown sugar

2 eggs

1 teaspoon vanilla extract

1 cup rolled oats, ground fine in a food processor

2 cups all-purpose flour

1 1/2 teaspoons salt

1/2 teaspoon baking soda

1 teaspoon baking powder

1/3 cup plain soy protein powder (optional)

2 1/4 cups chocolate chips

2 cups chopped walnuts

1/4 cup sweetened flaked coconut

Preheat the oven to 350°F.

Using an electric mixer, beat the butter in a bowl until it is light and fluffy. Add the two sugars and beat for about 30 seconds. Add the eggs and vanilla and beat to mix. Add the oats, flour, salt, baking soda, baking powder, and protein powder and mix until just combined. Stir in the chocolate chips, walnuts, and coconut with a wooden spoon.

Drop the dough by teaspoonfuls onto an ungreased cookie sheet. Bake for 15 minutes, rotating the cookie sheet on the oven rack once to ensure even browning. Remove the cookies from the baking sheet to cool on a wire rack.

Three Trans Fat–Free Piecrusts

Is there anything as lovely as a pie fresh from the oven topped with a flaky golden crown? Some piecrusts are just amazing—crisp and buttery with light, tender flakes that you can cut with a fork. And some crusts are awful—tough and stiff or soggy and pallid or dry and cracked. Many people wonder why they should go to the trouble of making a piecrust—and risking utter failure—when they can buy one at the market for a couple of bucks. The problem with store-bought crusts is that they are made with hydrogenated shortening, that is, trans fat. So, if you want to make a pie but you don't want to eat trans fat, you need to learn how to make a trans fat–free piecrust. The three versions that follow are perfect for all sorts of pies, from fruit to sweet to meat. Master these basic techniques and avoid the common mistakes and a perfect piecrust is just a few cups of flour away.

- Keep the butter or other fat very cold. Place the butter in the freezer for 20 minutes before starting to make the crust.
- Stir all of the dry ingredients together before adding the fats.
- Mix the dry ingredients and the fats quickly so the fats don't have a chance to soften or melt. A food processor is a wonderful tool for making piecrusts because the sharp blade blends the dry ingredients and the fats quickly, in just a few 10-second pulses. (Running the food processor instead of pulsing it may cause the mixture to come together in several small doughy balls, which may result in a tough, greasy crust.) If you don't have a food processor, use a pastry blender. As a last resort, use your fingers to blend the dry ingredients and the fats. Hold onto an ice pack to cool down the temperature of your hands, then dry them off and squeeze the dry ingredients and fats together quickly until the dough is pea-sized.

- Know when to stop mixing. When the dry ingredients and fats are combined, the mixture will resemble damp sand and take on a slightly yellow cast from the fat. There will be no large pieces of butter, lard, or coconut oil and the mixture will be dry and powdery.

- Add enough liquid to form the dough. If you use a food processor, remove the mixture from the bowl of the food processor and place it in a large bowl. (Never add liquid to the dry ingredients while the processor is running because it will be difficult to determine the proper amount.) Fill a measuring cup with very cold water. Use a tablespoon to sprinkle all of the water specified in your recipe over the mixture. Use your fingers or a fork to gather up the dough and start forming it into a ball. Sprinkle additional water over the dough and gather it gently with the spatula until it forms a cohesive mass. If you don't add enough water you'll have trouble rolling and shaping the crust later on. It is better to add too much water than too little.

- Let the dough rest. Flatten the dough into 2 disks, one slightly smaller than the other (the smaller disk will become the top crust). If the dough feels sticky, sprinkle a handful of flour over the top and bottom. Wrap the dough in plastic wrap and refrigerate it for at least 45 minutes or up to 2 days. Refrigerating the dough makes it easier to work with and keeps the fat cold. If you chill the dough for more than 3 hours, remove it from the refrigerator about 40 minutes before rolling it out.

- Use a quality rolling pin to roll out the dough. Basic wooden rolling pins with wooden handles on each end work well, as do tapered rolling pins without handles. Marble rolling pins tend to be heavy and awkward to use. Your work area should be a little higher than your waist so your elbows are bent and your palms rest on the work area.

- Use proper techniques to roll out the dough. On a counter or a flat table, sprinkle a cup of flour over a 15-inch square area. Dust your rolling pin with flour and place the dough in the center of the floured area. Starting in the center of the dough, apply gentle pressure with your rolling pin and roll the dough away from you. Pick up the dough, flip it over, and roll the other side the same way. Flip the dough over again and sprinkle your rolling pin and work area with additional flour. Holding the dough with one hand and your rolling pin in the other hand, roll from the center to the edges, rotating a quarter turn each time. Turn the dough over after every full rotation (use a metal spatula or dough scraper if needed) and add flour to the work area under the dough as needed. Flipping the dough keeps it from sticking to the work surface, incorporates more flour into the dough, and keeps the thickness even. If the edges seem to be cracking, brush them with a pastry brush dipped in water and press them together with your fingers. When the dough circle measures about 8 inches in diameter, it is too large to flip. Continue to roll it from the center to the edges, forming it into an even circle 12 to 13 inches in diameter and $1/8$ inch thick. Place your rolling pin in the center of the dough circle, pick up one side of the dough, and drape it over the rolling pin. Use the rolling pin to transfer the dough to the pie pan and gently press the dough down into the pan. Leave the edge hanging over the rim. Use the same technique to roll out the top crust, but only roll it to a size of 10 to 11 inches in diameter.

- Finish your pie. Add your filling to the bottom crust. Fruit fillings will shrink during baking, so can be piled high in the crust; potpie fillings should go to about $1/4$ inch below the rim of the pan. Brush the edges of your bottom crust with a pastry brush dampened with water. Use the rolling pin to transfer the top crust to the pie pan, laying it over the filling. Press the edges of the top and bottom crusts together with your fingers or a fork. Use scissors to trim away any excess dough from the edge. Form a fluted edge by pinching the dough between your thumb and forefinger and pressing in the center with the forefinger of your other hand, continuing all around the edge. Cut two 1-inch slits in the top crust to allow steam to escape while baking.

Common Piecrust Problems and Solutions

PROBLEM	SOLUTION
Dough is too cold or too warm.	Cold: Cover the dough in plastic wrap and leave at room temperature for 30 minutes. Warm: Do not reform the dough into a disk. Place it on a metal cookie sheet (using spatulas if needed) and refrigerate. Let the dough chill until firm, about 30 minutes.
Dough sticks to the work surface or rolling pin.	Carefully scrape the dough from the surface with a flat spatula or butter knife. Add more flour to the rolling pin and the work surface.
Dough develops large cracks during rolling.	The dough is too cold. Let it sit for 20 minutes at room temperature. Mend cracks by pressing the edges together, moistening slightly with a pastry brush dipped in cold water. Add a pinch of flour over the fixed area and roll out carefully.
Dough tears when being moved into the pie pan.	Moisten tears with a pastry brush dipped in cold water and press the edges together or patch with small pieces of dough.

Coconut Oil Piecrust

MAKES 2 (9-INCH) PIECRUSTS The combination of butter and coconut oil makes a flaky, puffy crust that will complement almost any sweet filling, particularly juicy fruit pies, such as blueberry or cherry. This rich and tender crust is wonderful for dishes that require only a top crust and can be used for the Apple Pocket Pies (page 89),or Lemon Buttermilk Pie (page 108). Because it is such a light and delicate pastry, it is too soft for cream pies and other desserts that require a prebaked pie shell.

In the bowl of a food processor fitted with a sharp blade, process the flour and salt. Add the butter and coconut oil and pulse until they are worked into the flour and no large pieces remain.

Remove the flour mixture to a bowl. Add the lemon juice and water and gather the dough together with your fingers or a fork to form a ball (add additional water as needed to bring the dough together into a cohesive mass). Divide the dough evenly into 2 balls and flatten each ball into a disk. Wrap the disks in plastic wrap and refrigerate for 1 hour.

On a lightly floured surface, roll one of the disks into a 12-inch round and place it in a 9-inch pie pan. Place your filling in the bottom crust and then roll out the remaining dough to make a top crust. Use the rolling pin to transfer the top crust to the pie pan, laying it over the filling. Press the edges of the top and bottom crusts together with your fingers or a fork. Use scissors to trim away any excess dough from the edge. Form a fluted edge by pinching the dough between your thumb and forefinger and pressing in the center with the forefinger of your other hand, continuing all around the edge. Cut two 1-inch slits in the top crust to allow steam to escape while baking. Bake according to the recipe instructions.

2^1/$_2$ cups all-purpose flour

1 teaspoon salt

^{1}/$_2$ cup cold unsalted butter, cut into small pieces

5 tablespoons coconut oil, at room temperature

2 teaspoons lemon juice

^{1}/$_4$ cup ice water

Lard Piecrust

MAKES 2 (9-INCH) PIECRUSTS A classic piecrust from back in the day. The most neutral-flavored lard, called leaf lard, is rendered from the fat around the kidneys of young pigs. It can sometimes be obtained from a butcher shop and rendered to make lard for pastry. If you don't happen to have rendered lard on hand, you can use the boxes of lard from the grocery store. But beware that most commercial lards contain "hydrogenated lard" (whatever that might be) and have a noticeable bacon flavor and aroma, making them unsuitable for most dessert pastries. The nice thing about lard is that it makes a flaky yet sturdy crust that is easy to roll out and transfer to the pie pan. Try this crust with Beef–Shiitake Mushroom Potpie (page 62) or Chicken-Tarragon Potpies (page 64).

2¹/₄ **cups flour**

¹/₂ **teaspoon baking powder**

¹/₂ **teaspoon salt**

¹/₂ **cup lard**

6 to 8 tablespoons cold water

In the bowl of a food processor fitted with a sharp blade, process the flour, baking powder, and salt. Add the lard and pulse until the mixture is the texture of cornmeal.

Remove the mixture to a bowl. Add 6 tablespoons of the water and gather the dough together with your fingers or a fork to form a ball (add additional water as needed to bring the dough together into a cohesive mass). Divide the dough evenly into 2 balls and flatten each ball into a disk. Wrap the disks in plastic wrap and refrigerate for 1 hour.

On a lightly floured surface, roll one of the disks into a 12-inch round and place it in a 9-inch pie pan. Place your filling in the bottom crust and then roll out the remaining dough to make a top crust. Use the rolling pin to transfer the top crust to the pie pan, laying it over the filling. Press the edges of the top and bottom crusts together with your fingers or a fork. Use scissors to trim away any excess dough from the edge. Form a fluted edge by pinching the dough between your thumb and forefinger and pressing in the center with the forefinger of your other hand, continuing all around the edge. Cut two 1-inch slits in the top crust to allow steam to escape while baking. Bake according to the recipe instructions.

PREBAKED PIECRUST: Preheat the oven to 425°F. Prepare and roll out the dough as instructed. Place the dough in two 9-inch pie pans. Prick the dough with a fork along the bottom and sides. Cover the dough surface with parchment paper and fill with pie weights. Bake for 10 minutes, lower the heat to 350°F and bake for 20 minutes more, or until the crust is golden brown. Remove the parchment paper and pie weights and allow the crust to cool before adding the filling.

Canola Oil Piecrust

MAKES 2 (9-INCH) PIECRUSTS Oil-based pie crusts can be heavy and dense, but for this one I use a French technique called *fraisage* to hydrate the flour proteins without toughening the dough. The tahini is optional, but it does improve the flavor of the crust. Rolling the dough between sheets of wax paper keeps it from tearing.

2 cups all-purpose flour

1 teaspoon salt

2 tablespoons tahini paste (optional)

$1/2$ cup canola oil

5 tablespoons cold water

In a large bowl, stir together the flour and salt and set aside. In a small bowl, stir together the tahini and oil with a fork. Add the water and stir. Add the tahini mixture to the flour mixture and combine with a few strokes of a wooden spoon. Gather the dough together with your fingers or a fork to form a ball (add additional water as needed to bring the dough together into a cohesive mass).

Divide the dough evenly into 6 pieces. Place a piece of the dough on a clean countertop and, using the heel of your hand, push on the dough as you slide it forward about 4 inches. Scrape up the piece of dough, set it aside, and repeat with the remaining dough until you've worked all of the dough. Reassemble the dough into a ball, divide it evenly into 2 balls and flatten each ball into a disk. Wrap the disks in plastic wrap and refrigerate for 30 minutes.

Wet your countertop with a damp sponge and cover it with a 12 by 16-inch sheet of waxed paper. Place one of the disks of dough on top of the waxed paper and top the dough with another sheet of waxed paper. Gently roll the dough into a 12-inch round and place it in a 9-inch pie pan. Place your filling in the bottom crust and then roll out the remaining dough to make a top crust. Use the waxed paper to transfer the top crust to the pie pan, laying it over the filling. Press the edges of the top and bottom crusts together with your fingers or a fork. Use scissors to trim away any excess dough from the edge. Form a fluted edge by pinching the dough between your thumb and forefinger and pressing in the center with the forefinger of your other hand, continuing all around the edge. Cut two 1-inch slits in the top crust to allow steam to escape while baking. Bake according to the recipe instructions

PREBAKED PIECRUST: Preheat the oven to 425°F. Prepare and roll out the dough as instructed. Place the dough in two 9-inch pie pans. Prick the dough with a fork along the bottom and sides. Cover the dough surface with parchment paper and fill with pie weights. Bake for 10 minutes, lower heat to 350°F and bake for 20 minutes more, or until the crust is golden brown. Remove the parchment paper and pie weights and allow the crust to cool before adding the filling.

Lemon Buttermilk Pie

MAKES 1 (9-INCH) PIE The slight tang of buttermilk along with the light whiff of lemon makes this pie an ideal accompaniment for blueberries or huckleberries. Although buttermilk is the main ingredient, this pie has a luscious sweet-tart flavor that is nothing like plain buttermilk. I like it served with almost any summer fruit, but it's irresistable served plain as well.

This is a good choice for summer entertaining as it travels well and is even better when prepared ahead of time and chilled. Bake it in the morning or the day before, then slice it and garnish with fresh berries.

1/2 recipe Coconut Oil Piecrust (page 103)

3 eggs, lightly beaten

1/4 teaspoon salt

2 tablespoons all-purpose flour

1 teaspoon finely grated lemon zest

2/3 cup sugar

1/4 cup unsalted butter, melted

11/4 cups buttermilk

2 teaspoons vanilla extract

Prepare and roll out a single piecrust according to the instructions on page 103. Place the piecrust in a 9-inch pie pan and trim and flute the edges. Prick the crust several times with a fork and refrigerate while you prepare the filling.

Preheat the oven to 375°F.

In a large bowl, whisk together the eggs, salt, flour, zest, and sugar. Whisk in the butter, followed by the buttermilk and the vanilla. Pour the filling into the prepared piecrust. Bake for 15 minutes, reduce the heat to 325°F, and bake for 30 minutes more, or until a knife inserted into the center of the pie comes out clean. Cool the pie on a wire rack for 1 hour before serving or refrigerate for several hours or overnight.

Rustic Plum Tart

SERVES 8 TO 10 This free-form tart can be made with any stone fruit, such as peaches, nectarines, apricots, or any variety of plum. It is especially pretty when made with a combination of purple, green, and yellow plums. The crust is tender, but sturdy enough to hold the juicy fruit.

To make the pastry: Using an electric mixer, combine the sugar, butter, vanilla, and cream cheese in a large bowl. Beat on medium for 2 minutes, or until light and fluffy. Add the egg and beat for 1 minute more. Add the flour and salt and blend on low for 1 minute, or until combined. Shape the dough into a ball, wrap it in plastic wrap, and freeze for 2 hours or refrigerate overnight.

Preheat the oven to 375°F. Lightly grease a large baking sheet.

To prepare the tart: Roll the dough out between two sheets of plastic wrap to a 15-inch circle with a thickness of $1/8$ inch. Remove the top layer of plastic wrap and transfer the dough to the prepared baking sheet. Remove the remaining plastic wrap. Arrange the plums on the dough, leaving a 3-inch border. In a small bowl, combine the jelly and 2 tablespoons of the water, and microwave for 1 minute, or until the jelly is melted. Brush the plums with the jelly. Fold the 3-inch border of dough over the plums (plums will be only partially covered). In a small bowl, beat the egg with the remaining 1 tablespoon water. Brush the dough with the egg wash. Sprinkle the dough with sugar.

Bake the tart for 30 minutes, or until the crust is light brown. Cool the tart on the baking sheet for 10 minutes, then use two spatulas to slide it onto a serving platter. Allow the tart to cool for 30 minutes more, then cut it into wedges and serve.

PASTRY

$1/2$ cup sugar

6 tablespoons unsalted butter, at room temperature

1 teaspoon vanilla extract

$1/2$ cup cream cheese

1 egg

2 cups all-purpose flour

$1/2$ teaspoon kosher salt

FILLING

10 to 12 medium plums, sliced thin

$1/4$ cup currant jelly

3 tablespoons water

1 egg

2 tablespoons sugar

Fresh Berry Tart

MAKES 8 TARTS These fat-free tart shells bake at a low temperature and become crispy little clouds of meringue. Pastry chefs often pipe the meringues through a pastry bag, but my method is much easier, requiring only a tablespoon. If you have a Silpat baking mat, pull it out for this recipe and skip the parchment paper.

TART SHELLS

4 egg whites

$^1/_2$ teaspoon cream of tartar

$^3/_4$ cup confectioners' sugar

1 teaspoon almond extract

FILLING

1 teaspoon vanilla extract

$^1/_4$ cup sugar

$1^1/_2$ cups sliced and chilled strawberries, blueberries, or raspberries

To make the tart shells: Preheat oven to 250°F.

Using an electric mixer, combine the egg whites and cream of tartar in a large bowl. Beat on medium until foamy, about 1 minute. Add the sugar $^1/_4$ cup at a time, beating after each addition. Then beat the mixture on high until stiff peaks form. Add the almond extract and beat for 10 seconds to combine.

Line a large baking sheet with parchment paper. Spoon a little blob of meringue at each corner to hold the parchment down. Use a tablespoon to make 8 mounds of meringue on the parchment. Use the back of the spoon to make a depression in the center of each mound. Bake for 90 minutes, or until the meringues are crisp and dry.

Cool the meringues on the pan for 5 minutes, then use a spatula to transfer them to a wire rack to cool completely. The tart shells taste best when used the same day, but they may be stored in a closed container for up to 2 days.

To make the filling: In a small bowl, toss the vanilla with the sugar. Sprinkle the sugar mixture over the berries.

To assemble the tarts: Place a generous spoonful of the berry mixture into each tart shell and serve immediately.

TROPICAL FRUIT TART: Prepare and bake the tart shells as instructed. Using an electric mixer, beat together 5 ounces softened lowfat cream cheese, 1 cup vanilla yogurt, 2 table-spoons honey, and 1 teaspoon lemon zest in a bowl. Cover and refrigerate for at least 1 hour. Spoon the filling into the tart shells, top with diced mango or papaya, and serve immediately.

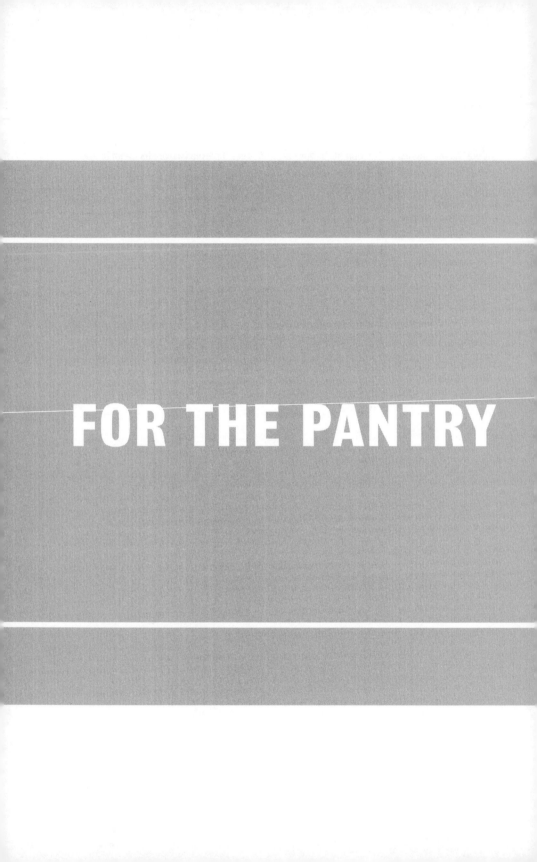

FOR THE PANTRY

Cindy B's Butter Blend

MAKES 2 CUPS Trying to reduce the cholesterol and saturated fat in your diet? You can eliminate the trans fat found in most margarines but keep the flavor of butter with this blend. Using canola oil adds monounsaturated fat, which helps increase your good cholesterol. The blend can be used as a spread for bread, toast, or pancakes and can be substituted for butter in most baked goods, such as muffins, breads, and scones. It's also great for cooking foods at medium to low temperatures, such as eggs or vegetables. Make this into a compound "butter" spread by blending in fresh chopped herbs, or add minced garlic for garlic bread.

$1/4$ cup buttermilk

$1/4$ cup cold water

1 teaspoon kosher salt

$1/2$ cup unsalted butter, at room temperature

$1/2$ cup canola oil

In a glass measuring cup, combine the buttermilk, water, and salt and stir to dissolve the salt. Set aside.

In the bowl of a stand mixer fitted with a whisk attachment, whisk the butter on medium for 30 seconds, or until the butter is very soft. With the mixer running, slowly drizzle in the canola oil. Stop the mixer 2 or 3 times to scrape down the sides and bottom of the bowl. When all of the canola oil is blended into the butter, drizzle in the buttermilk mixture and whisk until incorporated. Cover the bowl and refrigerate for at least 2 hours.

You can store the blend in a covered container, refrigerated, for up to 3 weeks.

Instant Oatmeal

SERVES 6 It's quick and easy to make individual servings of breakfast oatmeal. This recipe adds a touch of protein powder for extra nutrition. You can vary the fruit and spices—try dried pineapple with toasted coconut flakes, or chopped dates with toasted almond slivers—to add a new twist to breakfast.

In the bowl of a food processor fitted with a sharp blade, pulse the oats in four 10-second bursts, just enough to cut them slightly. Add the milk, protein powder, salt, brown sugar, cinnamon, raisins, and apple, and stir. Divide the oat mixture into six 1/2-cup portions and store in resealable plastic bags at room temperature for up to 1 year.

To prepare the oatmeal: Place 1 portion of the mix in a bowl and add 1 cup of hot water. Stir, then microwave on high for 2 minutes. (Use caution removing the bowl from the microwave, as it will be very hot.)

2 cups rolled oats

1/4 cup nonfat milk powder

3 tablespoons unflavored soy protein powder

1/2 teaspoon kosher salt

2 tablespoons brown sugar

1/2 teaspoon cinnamon

1/4 cup raisins

1/4 cup chopped dried apple

Homemade Cake Mix

MAKES 18 CUPS CAKE MIX; ENOUGH FOR 4 CAKES This versatile cake mix is convenient to have around the house to make a quick birthday cake or dessert. You can have a homemade cake baking in the oven within 15 minutes—and with no harmful trans fat. The basic mix makes a yellow cake, but with a few extra ingredients you can make spice cake, chocolate cake, or pineapple upside-down cake. For best results, allow the mix to sit at room temperature for 1 hour prior to mixing. If you use the mix straight out of your refrigerator, microwave it on low for 2 minutes to slightly soften the butter and coconut oil before using.

1 cup all-purpose flour

5 cups sugar

1/4 cup baking powder

1 tablespoon plus 1 teaspoon salt

1 (32-ounce) box cake flour

2 cups unsalted butter

1 cup coconut oil

In a very large bowl, blend the all-purpose flour, sugar, baking powder, and salt. In the bowl of a food processor fitted with a sharp blade, combine 3 cups of the cake flour and half of the butter. Process the mixture for about 1 minute, until it is fine in texture. Add the butter mixture to the all-purpose flour mixture. In the food processor, blend the remaining butter with 3 cups of cake flour and add it to the large bowl. Finally, in the food processor, blend the coconut oil and 3 cups of cake flour and add it to the large bowl. Add the remaining cake flour to the large bowl and stir the mixture well to combine all the ingredients.

Measure 4 1/2 cups of the cake mix into each of four 1-quart freezer bags. Store the mix in the refrigerator for up to 2 months or in the freezer for up to 6 months.

YELLOW CAKE: Preheat the oven to 325°F. Butter and flour a 9 by 13-inch cake pan or two 8-inch round pans.

In a large mixing bowl, place the contents of 1 bag of cake mix. In a small bowl, whisk together 2 eggs, 3/4 cup milk, and 2 teaspoons vanilla extract. Add 1 cup of the egg mixture to the cake mix. Using an electric mixer, beat for 2 minutes, or until fluffy and well combined. Scrape the sides of the bowl, add the remaining egg mixture, and beat for 1 minute more. Pour the batter into the prepared cake pan(s), smoothing it into an even layer.

Bake for 25 to 30 minutes, until the top is light golden brown and a skewer inserted into the center comes out clean.

Cool the cake on a wire rack for 5 minutes. Remove the cake from the pan and continue cooling on the rack for 1 hour before frosting. Frost with Chocolate Frosting (page 119) or Buttercream Frosting (page 120).

SPICE CAKE: Preheat the oven to 325°F. Butter and flour a 9 by 13-inch cake pan or two 8-inch round pans.

In a large mixing bowl, combine the contents of 1 bag of cake mix and 1 1/2 teaspoons cinnamon, 1/2 teaspoon ground ginger, 1/2 teaspoon ground cardamom, 1/8 teaspoon ground cloves, and 1/8 teaspoon ground nutmeg. In a small bowl, whisk together 2 eggs, 3/4 cup milk, 2 teaspoons vanilla extract, and 2 tablespoons molasses. Add 1 cup of the egg mixture to the cake mix. Using an electric mixer, beat for 2 minutes, or until fluffy and well combined. Scrape the sides of the bowl, add the remaining egg mixture, and beat for 1 minute more. Pour the batter into the prepared cake pan(s), smoothing it into an even layer.

Bake for 25 to 30 minutes, until the top is light golden brown and a skewer inserted into the center comes out clean.

Cool the cake on a wire rack for 5 minutes. Remove the cake from the pan and continue cooling on the rack for 1 hour before frosting. Frost with Buttercream Frosting (page 120).

CHOCOLATE CAKE: Preheat the oven to 325°F. Butter and flour a 9 by 13-inch cake pan or two 8-inch round pans.

In a large mixing bowl, combine the contents of 1 bag of cake mix and 1/2 cup cocoa powder. In a small bowl, whisk together 2 eggs, 1 cup milk, and 2 teaspoons vanilla extract. Add 1 cup of the egg mixture to the cake mix. Using an electric mixer, beat for 2 minutes, or until fluffy and well combined. Scrape the sides of the bowl, add the remaining egg mixture, and beat for 1 minute more. Pour the batter into the prepared cake pan(s), smoothing it into an even layer.

Bake for 25 to 30 minutes, until the edges of the cake pull away from the pan and a skewer inserted into the center comes out clean.

Cool the cake on a wire rack for 5 minutes. Remove the cake from the pan and continue cooling on the rack for 1 hour before frosting. Frost with Chocolate Frosting (page 119).

PINEAPPLE UPSIDE-DOWN CAKE: Preheat the oven to 325°F. Butter a 9 by 13-inch cake pan. Cover a baking sheet with aluminum foil.

In a large mixing bowl, place the contents of 1 bag of cake mix. In a small bowl, whisk together 2 eggs, 3/4 cup milk, and 2 teaspoons vanilla extract. Add 1 cup of the egg mixture to the cake mix. Using an electric mixer, beat for 2 minutes, or until fluffy and well combined. Scrape the sides of the bowl, add the remaining egg mixture, and beat for 1 minute more. Set aside.

Sprinkle 1/2 cup firmly packed brown sugar over the bottom of the prepared pan. Arrange the contents of a 20-ounce can of pineapple rings over the brown sugar. Place a maraschino cherry in the center of each pineapple ring. Pour the batter into the cake pan, smoothing it into an even layer over the pineapple rings.

Bake for 25 to 30 minutes, until the top is light golden brown and a skewer inserted into the center comes out clean.

Cool the cake on a wire rack for 5 minutes. Run a butter knife along the sides of the pan to loosen the cake's edges. Place the foil-covered baking sheet over the top of the pan and carefully flip the cake over. Remove the pan and continue cooling the cake on the rack for 1 hour before serving.

Chocolate Frosting

FROSTS 1 (8-INCH) LAYER CAKE OR 1 (9 BY 13-INCH) CAKE This is my all-time favorite chocolate frosting. It is light and satiny-smooth, and the sour cream balances out the chocolate. It's perfect for a yellow cake or a devil's food cake.

In a double-boiler over medium heat, melt the chocolate. Add the butter a few pieces at a time, stirring after each addition, until the butter and chocolate are completely melted and smooth. Remove the pan from the heat and let the mixture cool until it is just warm.

Using an electric mixer, beat together the confectioners' sugar, sour cream, and vanilla in a bowl. Add the chocolate mixture to the sugar mixture and beat on high for 3 to 4 minutes, scraping the sides of the bowl 2 to 3 times. The frosting should be shiny and thick. Spread over the cake using a long metal spatula.

5 ounces unsweetened chocolate

$1/2$ cup unsalted butter, cut into small pieces

$2^{1}/_{4}$ cups confectioners' sugar

1 cup sour cream

2 teaspoons vanilla extract

Buttercream Frosting

FROSTS 1 (8-INCH) LAYER CAKE OR 1 (9 BY 13-INCH) CAKE Perfect for spice cake or carrot cake, this is a basic frosting that is very quick and easy to make.

8 ounces cream cheese, softened

$1/2$ cup unsalted butter, at room temperature

2 cups confectioners' sugar

2 teaspoons vanilla extract

Using an electric mixer, beat together the cream cheese and butter until combined, about 1 minute. Add the sugar and vanilla and beat on high for 3 to 4 minutes, scraping the sides of the bowl 2 to 3 times. The frosting should be shiny and thick. Spread over the cake with a long metal spatula.

Cornbread Mix

MAKES 2 1/4 CUPS MIX; ENOUGH FOR 9 CORNBREAD SQUARES OR 12 MUFFINS It's convenient to have a mix around when you want a quick bread that you can pop in the oven to accompany dinner. This basic mix will make either cornbread or corn muffins. You can double or triple the recipe to make several mixes. When making the cornbread, just stir to combine and don't overmix the batter.

In a mixing bowl, stir together the cornmeal, flour, sugar, baking powder, and salt. Store the mix in a resealable plastic bag at room temperature for up to 1 year.

CORNBREAD: Preheat the oven to 375°F. Grease an 8-inch square baking pan.

Pour the mix into a bowl. Add 1 beaten egg, 1 cup milk, and 1/4 cup melted unsalted butter. Stir with a wooden spoon until smooth, about 1 minute. Pour the batter into the prepared pan.

Bake for 25 to 30 minutes, until a knife inserted in the center comes out clean. Cut the cornbread into 9 squares and serve warm.

CORNBREAD MUFFINS: Preheat the oven to 375°F. Grease a muffin tin. Prepare the batter as instructed above. Fill the muffin cups 2/3 full of batter. Bake for 15 to 20 minutes, until the muffins are light brown. Cool on a wire rack for 15 minutes, then remove the muffins from the tin and serve warm.

1 cup yellow cornmeal

1 cup all-purpose flour

1/4 cup sugar

1 tablespoon baking powder

1 teaspoon salt

Buttermilk Pancake Mix

MAKES 5 CUPS MIX (6 TO 8 PANCAKES PER CUP OF MIX) Need a short stack in a hurry? This mix is handy to have around your house or weekend cottage. Label it with the date you made it and the additional ingredients required. You can add dried blueberries or strawberries to the mix if desired.

4 cups all-purpose flour

3/4 cup powdered buttermilk

2 tablespoons baking powder

1 teaspoon baking soda

1 teaspoon salt

1/4 cup sugar

In a large bowl, whisk together the flour, buttermilk powder, baking powder, baking soda, salt, and sugar. Store in a covered container for up to 1 year.

BUTTERMILK PANCAKES: Heat a pancake griddle, a nonstick pan, or a well-seasoned cast-iron skillet over medium-high heat (about 350°F or until a few drops of water whiz around for several seconds before evaporating).

In a mixing bowl, whisk together 1 cup of the mix, 3/4 cup water, 1 egg, and 2 tablespoons of melted unsalted butter.

Brush the griddle with canola oil using a pastry brush. Spoon a small circle of batter onto the griddle as a test. Adjust the temperature if the test pancake is cooking too fast or too slow. Ladle the batter onto the griddle, about 1/4 cup per pancake, but don't allow the pancakes to run together. Pancakes should be turned once and only once. Wait until the top of each pancake is covered with air bubbles (4 to 5 minutes) then sneak a quick look underneath. If the lifted edge reveals a golden brown color, the pancake is ready to flip. While you're waiting for the second side to brown (4 to 5 minutes more), resist the compulsion to press the pancakes down with the spatula. Flattening the pancakes does not cook them any faster and it makes your pancakes less fluffy.

Place the pancakes in a single layer on a baking sheet and keep them uncovered in a warm oven while you cook the rest of the batter. Serve warm with lots of butter and maple syrup or fruit.

RESOURCES

I used several publications, books, and websites to develop the material for this book. If you want to dig deeper into trans fat or into the state of food manufacturing in general, I suggest this partial list of resources.

Center for Science in the Public Interest, including their excellent *Nutrition Action Health Letter.* www.cspinet.org/.

The work of Walter Willett, chairman of the Department of Nutrition at the Harvard School of Public Health, including his book, *Eat, Drink, and Be Healthy: The Harvard Medical School Guide to Healthy Eating.* New York: Simon & Schuster, 2001. For links to his other work: www.hsph.harvard.edu/faculty/WalterWillett.html.

The work of Mary Enig, including *Know Your Fats: The Complete Primer for Understanding the Nutrition of Fats, Oils, and Cholesterol.* Silver Spring, Maryland: Bethesda Press, 2000. For more on her research about trans fat, go to: www.enig.com/trans.html.

Eric Schlosser's *Fast Food Nation: The Dark Side of the All-American Meal.* Boston: Houghton Mifflin, 2001.

Fran McCullough's *The Good Fat Cookbook.* New York: Scribner, 2003.

The work of Marion Nestle, chair of the Department of Nutrition and Food Studies at New York University and her book *Food Politics: How the Food Industry Influences Nutrition and Health.* Berkeley: University of California Press, 2002.

The Wellness Letter, published by the School of Public Health at The University of California, Berkeley: www.berkeleywellness.com/.

EatingWell magazine: www.eatingwell.com/.

Consumer Reports magazine: www.consumerreports.org/main/home.jsp.

Bantransfats.com, Inc., a collection of links and references developed by a San Francisco lawyer who sued Kraft for selling Oreo cookies to children. (He dropped the lawsuit in the summer of 2003.)

ABOUT THE AUTHORS

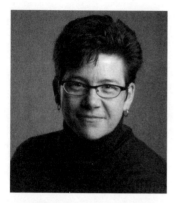

KIM SEVERSON writes about food for the *San Francisco Chronicle.* She was awarded the Casey Medal for Meritorious Journalism for her 2001 writing on childhood obesity and has won three James Beard Foundation journalism awards. She lives in Oakland, California.

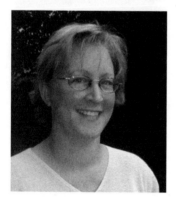

CINDY BURKE is a former chef who cooked at the Hunt Club and Place Pigalle in Seattle, Washington, and studied at the School for American Chefs in Northern California's Napa Valley. She often writes about food, organic farming, and nutrition. She lives in Seattle with her partner, Pat, and their daughter Allison.

INDEX

Food and Drug Administration (FDA),
     2, 11, 12–13
freezer staples
  fried chicken, 70
  pancakes, 83
  potpies, 65
  toaster waffles, 39
french fries, bistro, 53
fresh berry tart, 110–11
fries
  bistro french, 53
  herbed oven, 59
  nacho cheese, 87
frostings
  buttercream, 120
  chocolate, 119
fruit
  any-fruit-will-do scones, 37
  tropical, tart, 111

G

graham crackers, 80
granola, maple crunch, 34

H

herbed oven fries, 59
homemade cake mix, 116–18
homemade peanut butter, 84
hydrogenated/partially hydrogenated oil.
     See trans fat

I

ice cream sandwiches, 90–91
instant oatmeal, 115

J

jalapeño-cheddar poppers, 52

K

Kentucky Fried Chicken (KFC), 20
kid-friendly recipes
  apple pocket pies, 89
  fish sticks, crispy little, 86
  graham crackers, 80
  ice cream sandwiches, 90–91
  mini-pizzas, 88
  nacho cheese fries, 87
  pancakes, fluffy, 82–83
  parmesan chicken strips, 85
  peanut butter, homemade, 84
  teething biscuits, 81

L

labels. *See* nutrition labels
lamb, Cornish pasties with caramelized
     onions, potato and, 76–77
lard piecrust, 104–5
  in potpies, 62, 64
lasagne, roasted summer vegetable, 74–75
Legal Sea Foods, 26
lemon(y)
  buttermilk pie, 108
  -pepper crackers, 46
  yogurt muffins, 96

M

maple crunch granola, 34
McDonald's, 2, 7, 24
Meehan, Peter, 24
millet, in maple crunch granola, 34
mini-pizzas, 88
mixes
  butter blend, Cindy B's, 114
  buttermilk pancake, 122
  cake, homemade, 116–18
  cornbread, 121
  scone, 37
muesli, cinnamon-nut, 35
muffins
  cornbread, 121
  corn, roasted red pepper-cheddar, 58
  lemony yogurt, 96

N

National Academy of Sciences, 12
New England Journal of Medicine, 9
Newman, Nell, 24
Normann, William, 7
nutrition labels, 10–13
  reading, 15–17, 18–19

O

oats/oatmeal
  in chocolate chip cookies, 98
  in cinnamon-nut muesli, 35
  instant, 115
  in maple crunch granola, 34
  oatmeal-chocolate-cherry cookies, 97
  toasted oat tea biscuits, 56
obesity, 7, 9–10
old-fashioned popcorn, 48

Nutrition Facts (Wheat Crackers)

Serving Size 2 crackers (14 g)
Servings Per Container About 21

Amount Per Serving

Calories 60   Calories from Fat 15

	% Daily Value*
	2%
	0%
Total Fat 1.5g	
Saturated Fat 0g	
Polyunsaturated Fat 0.5g	
Monounsaturated Fat 0g	0%
...erol 0mg	3%
...10g	3%
	3%

Nutrition Facts

Serving Size 2 crackers (13 g)
Servings Per Container about 20

Amount Per Serving

Calories 70   Calories from Fat

	% Daily Value
Total Fat 3 g	5
Saturated Fat 1.5 g	8
Cholesterol 0 mg	0
Sodium 130 mg	5
Total Carbohydrate 8 g	3
Dietary Fiber less than 0 g	0
Sugars 1 g	
...in 1 g	

	Vitamin C 0
Vitamin A 0%	Iron 2

*Daily Values are based on a 2,000 calorie diet.
Values may be higher or lower based on your

	Calories:	2,000	2,500
	Less than	65g	80g
	Less than	20g	25g
	Less than	300mg	300mg
	Less than	2,400mg	2,400m
		300g	375g
		25g	30g

...T FLOUR (ENRICHED WITH NIACIN, IRON, THIA...
...FLAVIN, FOLIC ACID), COCONUT OIL, VEGETA...
...LY HYDROGENATED SOYBEAN AND COTTONS...
...USTARD SEED, DISTILLED VINEGAR, POPPY SEE...
...NING (AMMONIUM AND SODIUM BICARBONAT...
...MALTED WHEAT FLAKES, MALTED BARLEY FLO...
...ES... OWER SEEDS, MILLET, SESAME SE...
...AL FLAVOR.

Nutrition Facts (Cookies)

Serving Size 3 Cookies (32g)
Servings Per Container About 14

Amount Per Serving

Calories 160   Calories from Fat 70

	% Daily Value*
Total Fat 8g	12%
Saturated Fat 2.5g	12%
Cholesterol 0mg	0%
Sodium 105mg	4%
Total Carbohydrate 21g	7%
Dietary Fiber 1g	3%
Sugars 10g	
Protein 2g	

Vitamin A 0%	Vitamin C 0%
Calcium 0%	Iron 4%

* Percent Daily Values are based on a 2,000
calorie diet. Your daily values may be higher
or lower depending on your calorie needs:

	Calories:	2,000	2,500
Total Fat	Less than	65g	80g
Sat Fat	Less than	20g	25g
Cholesterol	Less than	300mg	300mg
Sodium	Less than	2,400mg	2,400mg
Total Carbohydrate		300g	375g
Dietary Fiber		25g	30g

INGREDIENTS: ENRICHED FLOUR (WHEAT
FLOUR, NIACIN, REDUCED IRON, THIAMINE
MONONITRATE (VITAMIN B1), RIBOFLAVIN
(VITAMIN B2), FOLIC ACID), SEMISWEET
CHOCOLATE CHIPS (SUGAR, CHOCOLATE,
DEXTROSE, COCOA BUTTER, SOY LECITHIN- AN
EMULSIFIER), SUGAR, PARTIALLY
HYDROGENATED SOYBEAN OIL, HIGH FRUCTOSE
CORN SYRUP, LEAVENING (BAKING SODA,
AMMONIUM PHOSPHATE), SALT, WHEY (FROM
...K), NATURAL...

MADE FROM: UNBLEACHED ENRICHED WHEAT
FLOUR, NIACIN, REDUCED IRON, THIAMIN
MONONITRATE (VITAMIN B1), RIBOFLAVIN
(VITAMIN B2), FOLIC ACID), MILK CHOCOLATE
(SUGAR, COCOA BUTTER, SKIM MILK POW...
CHOCOLATE LIQUOR, BUTTER OIL, SOY L...
SUGAR, PARTIALLY HYDROG...
ADDED AS AN EMULSIFIER, VANIL...
SHORTENING (SOYBEAN...
OILS), BUTTER, MA...
EGGS, BROWN...
SODA, TAP...

...R (WHEAT FLOUR,
...ONITRATE (VITAMIN
...LIC ACID), CRACKED
...ATED CANOLA AND
...Y (FROM MILK), SALT,

CO.

Nutrition Facts (Popcorn)

Serving Size: 2 Tbsp. (34g) Unpopped
(Makes 5 Cups Popped)
Servings Per Bag: 2.5 (About 12.5 Cup...

Amount/serving	As Pkgd/2 Tbsp. Unpopped	
Calories		1 C
Calories from Fat	120	
	50	

	%DV*	
Total Fat 5g	8%	1g
Sat. Fat 1g	5%	0g
Cholest. 0mg	0%	0mg
Sodium 320mg	13%	0mg
Total Carb. 20g	7%	25mg
Dietary Fiber 7g	29%	4g
Sugars 0g		1g
Protein 3g		0g
Vitamin A		<1g
Vitamin C	0%	
Calcium	0%	
Iron	0%	
	4%	

*Percent Daily Values are based on a 2,000 calorie diet. Your da...
values may be higher or lower depending on your calorie needs:

	Calories	2,000	2,500
Total Fat	less than	65g	
Sat Fat	less than		
Cholesterol			
Sodium			

...2,000
...higher
...needs;
...500
...0g
...25g
...300mg
...2400mg
...375g
...30g

...3%
...Fat 3g   3%
...3%
...5%
...10mg   0%
...80mg
...Carbohydrate 16g   3%
...Fiber 0g